Renal Failure in Paraplegia

Renal Failure in Paraplegia

by C. R. TRIBE, MA, DM, MCPath

Consultant Pathologist, Wycombe General Hospital,
High Wycombe, Bucks

Formerly, Senior Registrar in Morbid Anatomy,
Stoke Mandeville Hospital, Aylesbury, Bucks

With additional material
by J. R. SILVER, MB, BS, MRCP(Ed)

Consultant in Charge, Liverpool Regional Paraplegic Centre,
Promenade Hospital, Southport, Lancs

Postgraduate Lecturer in Surgery, Liverpool University

Formerly, Senior Research Assistant, National Spinal Injuries
Centre, Stoke Mandeville Hospital, Aylesbury, Bucks

London : PITMAN MEDICAL PUBLISHING COMPANY LIMITED

First published 1969

PITMAN MEDICAL PUBLISHING COMPANY LTD
46 Charlotte Street, London, W1

Associated Companies

SIR ISAAC PITMAN AND SONS LTD
Pitman House, Parker Street, Kingsway, London, W.C.2
P.O. Box 6038, Portal Street, Nairobi, Kenya

SIR ISAAC PITMAN (AUST.) PTY. LTD
Pitman House, Bouverie Street, Carlton, Victoria 3053, Australia

PITMAN PUBLISHING CORPORATION (S.A.) PTY. LTD
P.O. Box 7721, Johannesburg, Transvaal, S. Africa

PITMAN PUBLISHING CORPORATION
20 East 46th Street, New York, N.Y. 10017

SIR ISAAC PITMAN (CANADA) LTD
Pitman House, 381–383 Church Street, Toronto, 3

THE COPP CLARK PUBLISHING COMPANY
517 Wellington Street, Toronto, 2B

SBN: 272 79280 2

Printed in Great Britain at the Pitman Press, Bath
21 3614 11

Foreword

It was with great pleasure that I accepted the request of my colleagues Drs Tribe and Silver to write a short introductory note to their monograph *Renal Failure in Paraplegia*—a subject with which I have been concerned for many years.

Infection of the urinary tract resulting in chronic pyelonephritis and eventual renal failure is still the main killer of sufferers from spinal cord injury or disease. Therefore, prevention of this most serious complication remains a challenging problem to all concerned with the treatment and rehabilitation of paraplegia and tetraplegia. There is no doubt that the introduction of new concepts in the management of paraplegics and tetraplegics, in particular the treatment and prevention of pressure sores, has dramatically decreased the mortality rate of these patients in the acute and early stages and their duration of life is now vastly prolonged. However, the fact remains that renal failure with its effects on the cardiovascular system resulting from chronic infection of the urinary tract is still the main cause of late mortality in these patients. There are two reasons for this. In the first place, the initial treatment of the paralysed bladder is still all too often haphazard, especially in medical and surgical departments where knowledge, facilities, and staff are inadequate to deal competently with this most important complication of spinal cord injury. Once serious infection of the urinary tract has occurred in the acute and early stages following spinal paraplegia or tetraplegia, its definite eradication always remains doubtful in spite of all antibiotics and other therapeutic procedures so far available. Moreover, it has not been generally recognised that the dysfunction of the bladder itself resulting from spinal cord or spinal root damage may, by setting up changes in the anatomical structures, have adverse effects on ureters and kidneys, even in the presence of sterile urine. Second, the after-care, especially regular check-ups of paraplegics and tetraplegics following their discharge from accident, orthopaedic, neurosurgical, and even spinal units, is often still inadequate, where lack of communication between these units and the family doctor plays a significant part.

Since 1944, well over 4,000 paraplegics and tetraplegics, the majority of them of traumatic origin, have been treated at the National Spinal Injuries Centre, Stoke Mandeville. Thanks to the close co-operation which has existed through many years between the Centre and the Pathology Department of Stoke Mandeville Hospital, detailed autopsies have been performed on patients who died during the various stages of their paraplegia or tetraplegia. It was fortunate that Dr C. R. Tribe took a particular interest in the renal pathology of these post-mortem cases and he has made a careful and detailed histo-pathological study on 220 autopsies. In co-operation with Dr J. R. Silver, he has now written a comprehensive monograph in which the two authors analyse the pathological findings in the renal system in relationship to clinical data. On account of the histological pattern found in 174 cases, a division of pyelonephritis into four groups can now be suggested: (1) acute pyelonephritis; (2) acute complicating chronic pyelonephritis (complicating renal amyloidosis); (3) active chronic pyelonephritis; and (4) atrophic chronic pyelonephritis.

In their studies, the authors have paid particular attention also to the complex problems of amyloidosis and hypertension in chronic paraplegia, and this chapter will no doubt be of greatest interest to both clinicians and pathologists. The progress made in their studies of these complex biological problems is evident. However, it would be irrational to believe that they are solved. There still remains a wide field of investigation for those who want to contribute to the elucidation of these problems.

I am sure that this monograph will arouse great interest among those who are specially concerned with the study of the physiology and pathology of the urinary tract in spinal cord lesions and above all in the treatment and rehabilitation of paraplegics and tetraplegics.

Professor Sir Ludwig Guttmann

Preface

UNTIL THE INTRODUCTION of modern methods of treatment by D. Munro in 1936 and Sir Ludwig Guttmann in 1944, almost all patients with traumatic paraplegia died from acute ascending pyelonephritis and pressure sores within a year of injury.

With the advent of antibiotics, blood transfusion, and other modern methods of treatment, a large population of chronic paraplegics now exists. Although the immediate high mortality from acute pyelonephritis is now minimal, provided the principles of treatment laid down by Munro and Guttmann are followed, the majority of chronic paraplegics still die from causes directly related to their paraplegia. Renal failure accounts for three-quarters of these deaths, and is due to an interesting combination of chronic pyelonephritis, calculosis, amyloidosis, and secondary hypertension.

The sequelae of chronic paraplegia develop from two main causes. First, the muscular paralysis and loss of sensation lead to the development of pressure sores, osteomyelitis, and a high incidence of amyloidosis. Second, the impairment of bladder function leads to urinary sepsis and to back pressure on the kidney; these, combined with the stasis caused by immobility, lead to calculosis and chronic pyelonephritis. Secondary hypertension is often associated with chronic renal disease.

Although primarily affecting the renal tract, paraplegia produces changes throughout the body that are of interest to physicians and surgeons other than those immediately concerned with the treatment of paraplegia. The patients studied in this monograph were all treated and regularly observed at a Spinal Centre, so providing a unique opportunity to investigate the natural history of chronic pyelonephritis, amyloidosis, and secondary hypertension.

Part of the material in this monograph is derived from the author's thesis for the degree of Doctor of Medicine (Oxford) 1963 entitled *Post-mortem Findings in Paraplegic Patients*. This thesis was concerned with analysis of the necropsies performed on 150 patients who had died at the National Spinal Injuries Centre, Stoke Mandeville Hospital, England between 1945 and 1963, and dealt chiefly with the morbid anatomical changes in the urinary tract. These observations have been amplified in this monograph by a study of 70 further cases, making a total of 220. A detailed study of all the clinical notes provided the clinical and chronological background to the final pathological findings. The clinical data and histopathological material from such a large number of cases has made it possible to tabulate many analyses, often with an assessment of the incidence of different features.

Dr J. R. Silver, formerly Research Physiologist at Stoke Mandeville Hospital and now Physician in Charge of the Liverpool Regional Paraplegic Centre at Southport, has written the section on 'Diagnostic Tests for Urinary Tract Disease in Chronic Paraplegia'. He has also reviewed the whole text with the critical eye of a physician actively employed in the day-to-day management of paraplegics, and has added sections to the chapter on amyloidosis which describe the clinical and laboratory aspects of this disease.

C.R.T.

Definitions

PARAPLEGIA is derived from the Greek παραπληξία (a stroke on one side) and παραπλήσσειν (to strike at the side), and originally indicated the clinical condition now called hemiplegia. In modern pathological usage (*Shorter Oxford English Dictionary*), paraplegia is defined as, 'paralysis of the lower limbs and a part or whole of the trunk, resulting from an affection of some part of the spinal cord'. Quadriplegia means paralysis of all four limbs and the trunk.

The 220 necropsies were performed on patients with paraplegia and with quadriplegia but, for the sake of simplicity, the term paraplegia in this monograph covers both paralysis in the lower limbs and in all four limbs. Dietrick and Russi (1958) set a precedent for this terminology by combining cases of paraplegia and quadriplegia in their analysis of the autopsy findings in 55 paraplegic patients. The abbreviations paraplegics and quadriplegics will be used to indicate patients with paraplegia and quadriplegia.

In literature concerning paraplegia the levels of spinal cord injury are usually abbreviated as follows: C means cervical, T means thoracic, and L means lumbar. This practice will be followed in this monograph.

References

DIETRICK, R. B. and RUSSI, S. (1958) *J. Amer. Med. Ass.*, **166**, 41.

GUTTMANN, L. (1953) *Medical History of the Second World War. Surgery*, Ed. Z. Cope, pp. 422–516. London: H.M.S.O.

MUNRO, D. (1936) *J. Urol.*, **36**, 710.

Acknowledgements

WE OWE A special debt of gratitude to Sir Ludwig Guttmann who by his enthusiasm, original work, and example has been responsible for the modern treatment of paraplegia throughout Europe and the Commonwealth. He founded the National Spinal Injuries Centre, Stoke Mandeville, and has been the mentor of all doctors interested in paraplegia. We are grateful to him both for allowing us to study his patients, living and dead, and for his stimulus and interest without which this monograph would not have been written.

We also wish to thank Dr J. Walsh, the present Director, and all the medical staff at the National Spinal Injuries Centre, and Dr H. J. Harris and all pathologists, past and present, at Stoke Mandeville Hospital for their assistance and encouragement. For much meticulous work in the laboratory we should like to thank Mr W. A. Kears, Mr M. Casling, and their fellow technicians. For his un-flagging zeal and willingness in the post-mortem room, we wish to thank Mr E. Martin. Mr G. Standen and Miss Janet Plested have provided the excellent photographs and diagrams, and we also thank Mrs Keyna Avery and Mrs Myra Faulkner for all their secretarial assistance.

In addition, Dr J. R. Silver wishes to thank Mr N. O. K. Gibbon, Dr M. McConnell, Dr K. Wright and Dr H. J. Goldsmith for their assistance; the Liverpool University Photographic Department for the photographs; Miss Barbara Duckworth, Department of Surgery, Liverpool University, for the diagrams; Miss Kathleen Maglione and Mrs Christine Teale for their secretarial help; and the 'Action for the Crippled Child' for a grant.

Finally, we should like to thank most sincerely Dr J. R. Rawstron for reading the manuscript, correcting our English, and restraining our flights of fancy.

Contents

1

Historical Review

Not until early in the nineteenth century is the urinary tract at post-mortem examination of paraplegics described. Curling (1833, 1836) gave lucid descriptions of the results of infection on the urinary tract after paraplegia. He showed that the survival time after paralysis was proportional to the severity of infection, and mentioned the classical complications of calculi and paravesical abscesses.

In 1856 and 1858, William Gull, better known for his description of myxoedema, published details of thirty necropsies he had performed on paraplegic patients. Although he was primarily interested in the changes in the spinal cords of these patients, two of his descriptions of urinary tract pathology are worth quoting. The first concerned a man aged twenty who died three weeks after paraplegia due to 'myelitis'.

'The kidneys were large, the texture was soft and mottled by purulent infiltration into and amongst the tubules. The mucous membrane of the pelvis was congested and ecchymosed. The bladder was full of purulent and ammoniacal urine. Its lining membrane inflamed and sloughing.'

The second concerned a woman aged fifty with paraplegia due to 'degeneration of the cord.' Here he found, 'The cortical portions of both kidneys full of points of suppuration and the pelves and bladder were acutely inflamed.'

In 1889, Thorburn published *A Contribution to the Surgery of the Spinal Cord* which included some excellent descriptions of urinary tract pathology. One of these concerned the post-mortem findings in a man aged sixty-eight who had fallen from a ladder and lived for twenty-one days after a complete C.5 lesion. He described the urinary tract as follows—

The bladder contained a quantity of blood-stained turbid fluid, its mucous membrane hanging in shreds, beneath which the wall was dark and livid; inflammation had extended to the pelvic cellular tissue and the peritoneum. The kidneys were congested and presented numerous scattered points of suppuration; there was no dilatation of, nor suppuration in their pelves.

This is a description of acute haematogenous pyelonephritis secondary to severe cystitis. He also noted death due to exhaustion following very extensive bedsores, and quoted an example of bilateral acute haematogenous pyelonephritis with septicaemia and endocarditis of the aortic and mitral valves, a condition that still causes death in chronic paraplegics.

In the third edition of his *Textbook of the Principles and Practice of Medicine* (1891) C. H. Fagge gave a detailed and accurate description of the post-mortem findings in paraplegics. He stated that, 'in cases of this kind one finds the most intense cystitis and suppurative nephritis, and, indeed, these affections have most commonly been the direct cause of death'. Describing the kidneys he wrote, 'They are enlarged, intensely congested, and full of suppurating points and streaks, in other words they present all the characteristics of an ascending inflammation'.

Prior to this, Fagge (1876) described 244 cases of lardaceous disease and he attributed two of these to bedsores following fractures of the spine. In 1877 and 1885, Howship Dickinson devoted three chapters to lardaceous disease of the kidney in his *Textbook on Renal and Urinary Affections*. He quoted one case as being due to renal suppuration and calculi, and two cases to extensive chronic bedsores. These are the two major factors that lead to amyloidosis in chronic paraplegia. After these early references to amyloidosis in paraplegia there is a lapse of fifty-five years before modern writers have associated these two conditions and recognised the large part played by amyloidosis in the cause of renal failure in paraplegia.

By the turn of the century, the chief causes of death in chronic paraplegics had been described. These were renal failure due to ascending urinary infection, exhaustion due to bedsores, and amyloidosis due to a combination of the first two. The descriptions of the early writers illustrating the natural history of untreated paraplegia cannot be bettered. Nowadays, with chemotherapy and modern treatment based upon a better understanding of the patho-physiology of spinal cord injury, the septic sequelae of paraplegia do not invariably occur. If they do, death does not result for many years, so that hypertension secondary to renal disease has time to develop.

Between 1890 and 1920 the literature was mainly concerned with traumatic paraplegia due to injuries from gunshot wounds. It is ironic to note that, only with the advent of large numbers of these patients, especially following the First World War, was both the professional and public conscience about these helpless invalids first stimulated. Unfortunately, medical treatment of this period could do little to lengthen their brief survival.

Thompson Walker, writing in 1917 and 1937, stated that the most common, and usually fatal, complication in the paralysed bladder was infection. Of 339 patients with spinal injury admitted to the King George Vth Military Hospital from 1915–19, 160 (47·2%) died from urinary infection eight to ten weeks after. He further reported that 19 cases out of 111 (17·1%) died at the Star and Garter Home from urinary infection at a later stage, one to three years after injury. In 1937, Thompson Walker estimated the total mortality rate due to urinary sepsis in British soldiers with paraplegia in the First World War was 80 per cent. He referred to two types of pathology in these cases: (1) acute cystitis, often of the haemorrhagic type, leading to septic pyelonephritis —'a peculiarly fatal disease', 'these cases are either better in one week or dead'; and (2) chronic septic pyelonephritis with recurring acute pyelonephritis.

The American soldiers with paraplegia fared no better in this war. Frazier and Allen (1918) described 442 deaths in 717 cases (mortality rate 61·6%). Referring to the physical care of patients surviving the immediate effects of paraplegia, they put the prevention of bedsores of first importance, adding that, 'of greater significance is the probability of infection of the bladder, since sooner or later cystitis will be followed by ascending infection, pyelitis, pyonephrosis and death'. Connors and Nash (1934) and Kennedy (1946) say of the U.S. Army paraplegics that, 'fully 80 per cent of them die in the first few weeks in consequence of infection from bedsores and catheterisation'. French writers of this period tell the same story, and Wertheimer (1924) noted that, 'l'infection urinaire est constante et fatale'.

In the First World War patients with paraplegia due to gunshot wounds died as a result of catheterisation. Vellacott and Webb-Johnson (1919) alone appeared to realise this and produced by far the best mortality figures by avoiding catheterisation whenever possible.

The literature between 1920 and 1945 is chiefly devoted to the problem of how to treat the paralysed bladder without causing fatal ascending urinary tract infection. There are no reports of post-mortem studies on paraplegics in this period. Hinman (1938) discussed the treatment of the paralytic bladder in cases of spinal cord injury. He compared civilian with war injuries and stated, 'while fatalities are fewer, they mostly follow the same complications, namely urinary infection and bedsores on skin areas continually soiled by urine'. In 1943, Munro, the originator and great advocate of tidal drainage, concluded a paper on mortality in paraplegia by saying, 'death from genito-urinary sepsis would not be countenanced in my service'. Unfortunately, even today this ideal has not been reached.

This historical review shows that very few pathological studies on paraplegics had been made before 1945. The part played by urinary tract infection and pressure sores in the death of paraplegics was well recognised. It was not appreciated that, following the advent of antibiotics and modern therapy, chronic renal failure due to amyloidosis, pyelonephritis, and hypertension would become the main cause of death in chronic paraplegics.

Literature published subsequent to 1945 will be referred to and compared with our findings in the following chapters.

References

CONNORS, J. F. and NASH, I. E. (1934) *Amer. J. Surg.*, **26**, 159.

CURLING, T. B. (1833) *Lond. med. Gaz.*, **13**, 76.

CURLING, T. B. (1836) *Lond. med. Gaz.*, **18**, 325.

DICKINSON, W. H. (1877) *The Pathology and Treatment of Albuminuria*, 2nd ed., Chaps. 11–13. London: Longmans Green.

DICKINSON, W. H. (1877, 1885) *On Renal and Urinary Affections*. Parts II and III. London: Longmans Green.

FAGGE, C. H. (1876) *Trans. path. Soc. Lond.*, **27**, 324.

FAGGE, C. H. (1891) *Textbook of the Principles and Practice of Medicine*, 3rd. ed., Vols. I and II. London: J. & A. Churchill.

FRAZIER, C. H. and ALLEN, A. R. (1918) *Surgery of the Spine and Spinal Cord*. New York: Appleton.

GULL, W. (1856) *Guys Hosp. Reports*, **2**, 143.

GULL, W. (1858) *Guys Hosp. Reports*, **4**, 169.

HINMAN, F. (1938) *Surgery*, **4**, 649.

KENNEDY, R. H. (1946) *Ann. Surg.*, **124**, 1057.

MUNRO, D. (1943) *J. Amer. Med. Ass.*, **122**, 1055.

THOMSON WALKER, J. (1917) *Lancet*, **i**, 173.

THOMSON WALKER, J. (1937) *Brit. J. Urol.*, **9**, 217.

THORBURN, W. (1889) *A Contribution to the Surgery of the Spinal Cord*. London: Chas. Griffin.

VELLACOTT, P. N. and WEBB-JOHNSON, A. E. (1919) *Lancet*, **i**, 733.

WERTHEIMER, P. (1924) *Lyon Chir.*, **21**, 309.

2

The Causes of Death in Chronic Paraplegia

BEFORE PROCEEDING to an analysis of renal failure in chronic paraplegia it is essential to look briefly at the chief causes of death in chronic paraplegics. Only with this knowledge will the part played by renal disease be seen in proper perspective.

In a previous analysis of the causes of death in paraplegia (Tribe, 1963a; 1963b) it was pointed out that the 150 necropsies studied represented only about 40 per cent of the total deaths after admission to the National Spinal Injuries Centre. The addition of a further 70 cases, making a total of 220 necropsies studied, amplifies the previous work and provides a reasonable survey of the causes of death in paraplegics. Since this monograph is concerned mainly with renal failure in chronic paraplegia, comparison of the findings in this series with those in other modern series will chiefly be confined to the renal aspect of the pathological findings.

Division of Cases

In order to break down the cases into groups which could be compared three primary divisions were made.

I. DURATION OF PARAPLEGIA—ACUTE AND CHRONIC

Those patients dying within the first three months of paralysis had basically different causes of death from those dying subsequently. In accordance with previous experience (Tribe, 1963a; 1963b), a primary division of the cases has therefore been made into Acute and Chronic Paraplegics.

II. CAUSE OF PARAPLEGIA—TRAUMATIC AND NON-TRAUMATIC

Surprisingly, this division has proved to be of only little value. Unless the aetiology of the paraplegia leads to death *per se* (e.g. malignant disease), it appears to play little part in the ultimate cause of death. In later chapters these two groups will usually be considered together.

III. RELATION OF DEATH TO PARAPLEGIA—RELATED AND NON-RELATED

This division is important and was made on the following criterion often required for medico-legal reasons—'Had this patient not been a paraplegic would he have died?' This division was made according to the primary cause of death. In many of the patients dying from causes unrelated to paraplegia there were significant and contributory pathological processes that were related to paraplegia. These will be discussed later where relevant. For example, one chronic paraplegic placed in the traumatic unrelated group died from peritonitis due to perforation of a gastric ulcer. His early renal failure due to pyelonephritis and amyloidosis resulting from his paraplegia, did not alter his allotment to this group as this was not the primary cause of death.

The 220 cases can now be divided as in Table 2.1.

TABLE 2.1
Classification of Paraplegia

ACUTE PARAPLEGIA	Death within three months of paralysis	
	46 cases	
Group I. Death related to paraplegia		33 cases
Group II. Death unrelated to paraplegia		13 cases
CHRONIC PARAPLEGIA	Death more than three months after paralysis	
	174 cases	
(a) *Traumatic cases* (Paraplegia due to trauma, including gunshot wounds)		
	123 cases	
Group A. Death related to paraplegia		97 cases
Group B. Death unrelated to paraplegia		26 cases
(b) *Non-traumatic cases* (Paraplegia due to causes other than trauma)		
	51 cases	
Group C. Death related to paraplegia		20 cases
Group D. Death unrelated to paraplegia		31 cases

These groups, which are important for a full understanding of the findings in this post-mortem series, can be abbreviated in the following diagram—

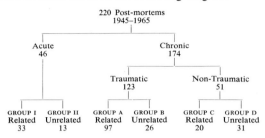

220 Post-mortems
1945–1965

Acute
46

Chronic
174

Traumatic
123

Non-Traumatic
51

GROUP I
Related
33

GROUP II
Unrelated
13

GROUP A
Related
97

GROUP B
Unrelated
26

GROUP C
Related
20

GROUP D
Unrelated
31

Groups I and II (Acute Paraplegia: Death Within Three Months of Paralysis—46 Cases)

Most deaths related to paraplegia were due to massive pulmonary embolism (16 cases) discussed by Walsh and Tribe (1965), and respiratory failure in high cervical lesions (12 cases). The high mortality among patients with high cervical injuries has been found in other series. Wolman (1965) described 30 patients who died within eleven days of sustaining a traumatic quadriplegia, and Silver (1968) described 5 patients who died within eighteen days of injury. At post-mortem, severe pulmonary oedema without any inflammatory reaction was the most common finding.

The patient with a high cervical injury maintains ventilation almost entirely with his diaphragm, although a little assistance is obtained from his auxiliary muscles of respiration. The vital capacity is consequently greatly reduced and, when the diaphragm is also involved, vital capacities as low as half a litre have been recorded (Guttmann and Silver, 1965). The ventilatory capacity is further reduced by the high incidence of aspiration pneumonia, head injury, and associated injuries, particularly fractures of the sternum and ribs. This results in a progressive increase in the dead space of the lungs. When the patient's tidal air equals his dead space, carbon dioxide retention and anoxia supervene and the patient dies unless he is placed in a respirator.

In the unrelated group, 10 out of the 13 patients died from associated traumatic injuries. No further analysis of these patients is needed except to note that none died from renal failure, and only 12 out of the 46 had clinical and laboratory evidence of urinary infection during life. Of the 43 cases in which kidney histology was available only two showed evidence of pyelonephritis. This is in dramatic contrast to the picture before 1945 (Chapter 1). These figures augur well for the future prognosis of paraplegics and there is no doubt, from clinical observations since the Second World War, that the life expectancy of paraplegics is steadily improving (Guttmann, 1962).

In recent years a much greater number of acute paraplegics, especially those with cervical lesions, have been admitted to Stoke Mandeville Hospital. Thus, 42 out of the 46 acute paraplegics in this series were admitted between 1958 and 1965. The majority of the chronic paraplegics in this series, however, were first admitted before 1958. Urinary infection occurred in all these patients and its effects played a predominant part in their death.

Groups A, B, C and D (Chronic Paraplegia: Death More than Three Months after Paralysis—174 Cases)

GROUP A (CHRONIC TRAUMATIC PARAPLEGIA: DEATH RELATED TO PARAPLEGIA—97 CASES)

A summary is shown in Table 2.2.

Comments on Primary Causes of Death in Group A

1. Renal failure was by far the most common primary cause of death in this group and will be discussed in the subsequent chapters.

2. Of the 7 fatal cases of cerebral haemorrhage, 6 patients had hypertension which was presumed secondary to chronic renal disease that had developed after paraplegia. These will be discussed in the chapter on Hypertension in Chronic Paraplegia.

The seventh case occurred in a forty-two year old man who had a incomplete traumatic paraplegia at C.6 for fourteen years. Two years before death he had a nephrectomy for severe, unilateral, acute on chronic renal infection. Subsequently, his urine remained sterile and at no time was there any clinical evidence of hypertension. His death followed a transient hypertension which developed after a prostigmine fertility test (Guttmann, 1953). At the post-mortem there was no pathological evidence of hypertension to account for the gross cerebral haemorrhage, and the remaining kidney was free from pyelonephritis. Amyloidosis, of mild degree, had not involved the cerebral vessels. Bors (1955) reported a similar case of a quadriplegic who died from a sub-arachnoid haemorrhage due to paroxysmal hypertension precipitated by an enema. Paroxysmal hypertension occurring in patients with paraplegia above T.5 will be discussed in Chapter 7.

3. Persistent chronic infection of the bladder appears to be related to carcinoma in paraplegics (Kawaichi, 1960; Tribe, 1963b; and Melzak, 1966) and this will be discussed in Chapter 5.

4. Three patients were considered to have died from toxaemia due to extensive pressure sores. In all 3 the bedsores were acute and gross, and the overwhelming infection caused death before treatment

TABLE 2.2

Group A (Chronic traumatic paraplegia: Death related to paraplegia—97 cases)

AVERAGE AGE AT DEATH   40·9 years

Aged up to 30	12 cases
Aged 30–39	40 cases
Aged 40–49	26 cases
Aged 50 and above	19 cases

AVERAGE SURVIVAL TIME AFTER PARAPLEGIA   10·0 years

LEVELS OF PARAPLEGIA	COMPLETE	INCOMPLETE	TOTAL
Cervical	11	10	21
Thoracic 1–4	6	0	6
Thoracic 5–8	19	1	20
Thoracic 9–12	32	3	35
Lumbar and Cauda Equina	6	9	15

PRIMARY CAUSE OF DEATH	NO OF CASES
1. Renal failure	69
2. Cerebral haemorrhage	7
3. Carcinoma of bladder	3
4. Toxaemia from pressure sores	3
5. Septicaemia and ulcerative endocarditis	3
6. Meningitis	2
7. Post-operative shock	2
8. Lung abscess	1
9. Respiratory failure in cervical lesions	6
10. Cerebral abscess	1

could be effective. None developed amyloidosis. Toxaemia from pressure sores is now extremely rare as a direct cause of death in paraplegics treated at spinal centres. However, it will be shown that pressure sores and underlying osteomyelitis are the chief causes of amyloidosis which is so largely concerned in the renal failure of chronic paraplegia.

5. In 3 patients, septicaemia with acute ulcerative endocarditis was the major cause of death. In 2 of these, the source of the infection was the kidneys and there was chronic pyelonephritis with terminal acute necrotising papillitis (Fig. 2.1). In the third patient, the acute haemolytic streptococcal endocarditis of all four heart valves apparently originated from gross

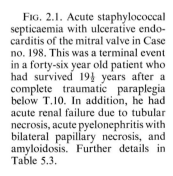

FIG. 2.1. Acute staphylococcal septicaemia with ulcerative endocarditis of the mitral valve in Case no. 198. This was a terminal event in a forty-six year old patient who had survived 19½ years after a complete traumatic paraplegia below T.10. In addition, he had acute renal failure due to tubular necrosis, acute pyelonephritis with bilateral papillary necrosis, and amyloidosis. Further details in Table 5.3.

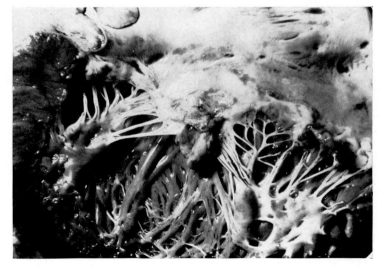

pressure sores. This patient is of special interest and his case history is included in Chapter 6 (p. 74).

Details of 3 further cases of septicaemia and endocarditis causing death in chronic paraplegics were available. (One of these is included in the non-traumatic Group C; one, who died in chronic renal failure, had an acute endocarditis superimposed upon old rheumatic disease of the mitral valve, and one case has been studied by Dr J. R. Silver at Southport). It is notable that 5 of these 6 cases had generalised amyloidosis (severe in 4 of them) and this suggests that natural resistance to infection is modified in some way by amyloid disease. This will be discussed further in the chapter on Amyloidosis (p. 61).

6. One case of meningitis was due to direct extension of a perivesical abscess following renal suppuration. The other followed invasion of the spinal canal by an epithelioma arising in a chronic pressure sore.

7. Two patients died from shock after operation —nephrolithotomy in one instance, and the formation of an ileal bladder in the other. Both operations were performed for urinary complications of paraplegia.

8. The patient who died from a lung abscess is of special interest. He was a man aged seventy who had survived for thirty-seven years after a gunshot wound in the First World War had produced an incomplete paraplegia at T.7. Post-mortem examination revealed how chronic urinary tract infection finally caused his death. A large calculus had formed in the first part of the right ureter, and was associated with severe chronic pyelonephritis. The calculus had ulcerated through the ureteric wall producing a perinephric abscess which had extended further to form a right sub-phrenic abscess. This abscess had then perforated through the diaphragm to cause a large lung abscess in the lower lobe of the right lung. He died from a massive haemoptysis.

The dotted line at this stage in Table 2.2 indicates that the deaths in sub-groups 9 and 10 were peculiar in being related both to their level of injury (cervical) and their paraplegia.

TABLE 2.3

Group B (Chronic traumatic paraplegia: Death unrelated to paraplegia—26 cases)

AVERAGE AGE AT DEATH	46·0 years		
	Aged up to 30	5 cases	
	Aged 30–39	5 cases	
	Aged 40–49	5 cases	
	Aged 50 and above	11 cases	

AVERAGE SURVIVAL TIME AFTER PARAPLEGIA   9·4 years

LEVELS OF PARAPLEGIA	COMPLETE	INCOMPLETE	TOTAL
Cervical	1	2	3
Thoracic 1–4	1	1	2
Thoracic 5–8	6	0	6
Thoracic 9–12	6	0	6
Lumbar and Cauda Equina	3	6	9

PRIMARY CAUSE OF DEATH	NO OF CASES
1. Coronary heart disease	6
2. Pulmonary infection	4
3. Abdominal catastrophe	3
4. Malignant disease	3
5. Post-operative shock	2
6. Other causes—	
Focal glomerulonephritis	1
Dissecting aneurysm	1
Cirrhosis of the liver	1
Pulmonary tuberculosis	1
Gastro-enteritis	1
Agranulocytosis	1
Cerebral haemorrhage	1
Hypertensive heart disease	1

Some comment on the 21 cervical cases in Group A is relevant at this stage. Fourteen showed a similar age and disease pattern as the thoraco-lumbar cases—viz. 10 cases of renal failure and one each of cerebral haemorrhage, carcinoma of the bladder, septicaemia and ulcerative endocarditis, and post-operative shock.

9. Of the remaining patients, 6 were classified as dying from respiratory failure. Two were elderly patients who died from bronchopneumonia, one at nine months and one at a year after paralysis. Their bronchopneumonia was undoubtedly exacerbated by the paralysis of their chief expiratory muscles. The cervical patient is always prone to develop an aspiration pneumonia. Another 2 patients died from acute pulmonary oedema associated with 'flare-ups' of unilateral pyelonephritis at $3\frac{1}{4}$ and $4\frac{1}{4}$ years after paralysis. The last 2 patients had further upward extension of the traumatic lesions of their cervical spinal cords, leading to respiratory failure at $1\frac{1}{2}$ and fourteen years after paralysis respectively. This is in keeping with the findings of Barnett *et al.* (1966), who reported 8 patients out of 591 traumatic paraplegics who developed the late onset of a progressive myelopathy in the cervical region. These findings suggest that the survival time of chronic cervical paraplegics is less predictable than thoraco-lumbar cases, and that in both the acute and chronic stages the prognosis of quadriplegics is uncertain.

10. The patient in this group is unique. He was a man aged seventy-two with complete paraplegia below C.7 after a car accident. He was treated in another hospital with traction to his spine by skull calipers. After four months he suddenly developed signs of a right hemiparesis and aphasia, thought to be due to cerebral thrombosis. There were no clinical signs of increased intracranial pressure. At post-mortem it was found that one of the burr holes made for the skull traction had penetrated through an abnormally thin skull bone, and allowed infection to enter the skull with the formation of a large chronic cerebral abscess $2\frac{1}{2}$ in. in diameter in the left temporal lobe.

GROUP B (CHRONIC TRAUMATIC PARAPLEGIA: DEATH UNRELATED TO PARAPLEGIA—26 CASES)

A summary is shown in Table 2.3.

Comment

This group comprises cases where the primary causes of death were not directly related to paraplegia. Discussion of the more debatable aspects of this selection is included in the comments on Group D, Table 2.6 (p. 9).

Many of these patients also suffered from infective complications of their paralysis which contributed to death. Of the 26 patients, 21 had chronic urinary infection, and from the sections of the 23 kidneys that were available for histological examination 4 showed severe, 4 moderate, and 8 slight pyelonephritis; only 7 kidney sections showed no evidence of infection.

Four patients had amyloidosis at death. In one this was almost certainly secondary to spinal and pulmonary tuberculosis, but in the other 3 early renal failure from amyloidosis had contributed to death, and was due to the septic complications of paraplegia. The primary causes of death in these 3 patients were myocardial infarction, peritonitis due to perforated peptic ulcer, and multiple cerebral thromboses—none directly related to paraplegia.

There were 51 cases of non-traumatic chronic paraplegia (Groups C and D) and the causes of paraplegia are listed in Table 2.4.

TABLE 2.4

Groups C and D (Paraplegia due to non-traumatic causes)

CAUSE OF PARAPLEGIA		NO OF CASES
Primary tumours of the spinal cord		13
Glioma	4	
Ependymoma	3	
Haemangioma	3	
Chordoma	1	
Neurofibroma	1	
Medulloblastoma	1	
Transverse myelitis		12
Metastatic tumours		6
Carcinoma of lung	3	
Carcinoma of prostate	1	
Neuroblastoma	1	
Hodgkin's disease	1	
Vascular lesions of the spinal cord		4
Prolapsed intervertebral disc		4
Disseminated sclerosis		3
Osteomyelitis		2
Poliomyelitis		2
Spina bifida		1
Chronic meningitis		1
Epidural abscess		1
Tuberculosis of the spine		1
Following aortogram for investigation of malignant hypertension		1
		51

GROUP C (CHRONIC NON-TRAUMATIC PARA-
PLEGIA: DEATH RELATED TO PARAPLEGIA—
20 CASES)

A summary is shown in Table 2.5.

Comments

The similarity between this group and the non-
cervical cases in Group A (Table 2.2, p. 5) is

primary causes of death in Groups B and D, elabor-
ated in Tables 2.3 and 2.6.

There is no evidence to suggest that paraplegia
predisposes to coronary heart disease, and this will
be discussed further in the chapter on Hypertension
in Chronic Paraplegia.

Some authors (Dietrick and Russi, 1958; Caravati
et al., 1958) regard cirrhosis of the liver as a common

TABLE 2.5

Group C (Chronic non-traumatic paraplegia: Death related to paraplegia—20 cases)

AVERAGE AGE AT DEATH	39·7 years		
	Aged up to 30	2 cases	
	Aged 30–39	9 cases	
	Aged 40–49	5 cases	
	Aged 50 and above	4 cases	

AVERAGE SURVIVAL TIME AFTER PARAPLEGIA	9·3 years		
LEVELS OF PARAPLEGIA	COMPLETE	INCOMPLETE	TOTAL
Thoracic 1–4	3	0	3
Thoracic 5–8	4	2	6
Thoracic 9–12	8	2	10

Plus one case of Poliomyelitis in which the level of the lesion was unrecorded.

PRIMARY CAUSES OF DEATH	NO OF CASES
Renal failure	17
Carcinoma of the bladder	1
Post-operative shock	1
Septicaemia and ulcerative endocarditis	1

evident. It appears that if death is related to paraplegia, the cause of the paraplegia, whether traumatic
or non-traumatic, plays no part either in the major
cause of death or the overall survival time. The only
exception appears to be the traumatic cervical group
in which causes of death and prognosis are more
variable. The only comment in this group is that the
patient who died from post-operative shock had
nephrolithotomy performed on his one surviving
kidney.

GROUP D (CHRONIC NON-TRAUMATIC PARA-
PLEGIA: DEATH UNRELATED TO PARAPLEGIA
—31 CASES)

A summary is shown in Table 2.6.

Comment

The primary causes of death in this group are
similar to those in Group B, the only difference being
a much shorter survival time in the non-traumatic
group, related to the higher incidence of malignant
disease.

Some further comments are needed concerning
the possible relationships to paraplegia of the

cause of death in paraplegics. Of the 4 cases of
hepatic failure in these two groups, 3 died from
complications of post-necrotic cirrhosis which
developed after their paraplegia. In contrast to other
authors, they were included in the unrelated group
as their cirrhosis apparently developed independently of blood transfusions or other treatment
related to their paraplegia. This selection is debatable, and the recent epidemics of infective hepatitis
in hospitals associated with renal dialysis pro-
grammes has focussed attention on the risks to both
medical staff and patients. This hospital-acquired
disease carries a high mortality, 1:8, and is not
necessarily transmitted by blood but may be transmitted by blood contaminated needles or even
through skin abrasions (leading articles, *Brit. Med.
J.*, April 1966, p. 997; August 1966, p. 426).

The 10 patients in the two groups who died from
bronchopneumonia and pulmonary infection did
not have quadriplegia. However, even in patients
with mid-thoracic injuries the paralysis of the abdominal muscles diminishes the vital capacity and
impairs the patient's ability to cough, so that secre-
tions drain down to the lowermost parts of the lungs

TABLE 2.6

Group D (Chronic non-traumatic paraplegia: Death unrelated to paraplegia—31 cases)

AVERAGE AGE AT DEATH   45·0 years

Aged up to 30	6 cases
Aged 30–39	5 cases
Aged 40–49	7 cases
Aged 50 and above	13 cases

AVERAGE SURVIVAL TIME AFTER PARAPLEGIA   4·8 years

LEVELS OF PARAPLEGIA	COMPLETE	INCOMPLETE	TOTAL
Cervical	3	1	4
Thoracic 1–4	3	1	4
Thoracic 5–8	5	2	7
Thoracic 9–12	10	2	12
Lumbar and Cauda Equina	1	1	2

Plus poliomyelitis, 1 case, and level unrecorded, 1 case.

PRIMARY CAUSE OF DEATH		NO OF CASES
1. Malignant disease		12
Carcinomatosis	7	
Involvement of brain stem by spinal cord tumours	5	
2. Bronchopneumonia		6
3. Coronary heart disease		4
4. Hepatic failure		3
5. Renal failure unrelated to paraplegia		2
6. Meningitis		2
7. Acute displacement of posterior mediastinum		1
8. Suicide		1

and the patients may develop aspiration pneumonia. The striking relationship between the incidence of pneumonia and the level of the spinal cord injury is borne out by the observation that, in a series of 50 traumatic paraplegics at the Liverpool Regional Paraplegic Centre, 18 were either admitted with pneumonia or developed pneumonia during the early stages of treatment. The posterior basal segments of the lungs were always involved. Of the 29 patients with cervical injuries, 12 developed this type of pneumonia, compared with 5 out of 15 thoracic patients and only one out of 6 patients with lumbar lesions (Silver, 1968).

The two patients with renal failure in Group D are of interest. The first died in acute uraemia and was diagnosed at post-mortem as acute pyelonephritis. Microscopy of the kidneys, however, revealed an acute focal glomerulonephritis of unknown aetiology. The second, a man aged forty-six, developed a complete paraplegia below T.9 following a diagnostic aortogram for severe hypertension. Four years later he died from renal failure due to malignant hypertension with no evidence of recent pyelonephritis. (Further details are given on p. 97.)

Although the survival time of the patients in this group was 4·8 years as compared to 9·4 years in Group B, pathological study revealed a similar pattern of renal disease derived from the infective complications of paraplegia. Of the 31 patients, 26 had chronic urinary infection. Histological examination of the kidneys showed changes of pyelonephritis in 19 (2 severe, 9 moderate, and 8 slight). Only 11 patients had no evidence of infection in their kidneys.

Two patients had amyloidosis at death. One man, aged forty at the time of death, had survived fourteen years after an incomplete cauda equina lesion from neurological complications of beri-beri that he developed as a prisoner of war in Singapore. He had persistent pressure sores for many years and finally died from an overwhelming lung infection. His blood urea was normal. Microscopy revealed a moderate degree of generalised amyloidosis with only early involvement of the kidneys. The second, who will be described in detail in Chapter 6, on Amyloidosis, was a young girl who had no pressure sores and only mild urinary infection, and yet she died with gross amyloidosis apparently related to a huge thoracic neuroblastoma.

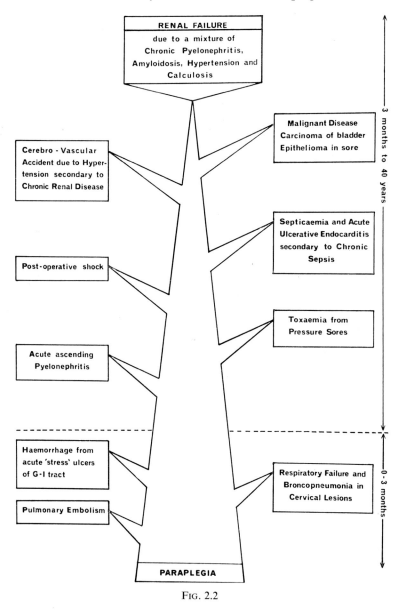

FIG. 2.2

Summary

In the first three months after sustaining a traumatic injury to the spinal cord, resulting in a partial or complete paraplegia, a patient may die of injuries acquired at the same time as the spinal injury, from pulmonary embolism, or, in the case of a cervical injury, from respiratory failure.

Once he has survived three months after the spinal injury there is little difference between the natural history of his condition whether it be due to trauma or other diseases causing a similar degree of paralysis, unless the paraplegia is due to metastatic carcinoma.

The paralysis and loss of sensation renders him liable to develop pressure sores, and paralysis of his bladder leads to the ascent of infection to his kidneys. These two factors lead to chronic renal failure and death in 75 per cent of chronic paraplegics, from a combination of pyelonephritis, calculosis, amyloidosis, and secondary hypertension.

These changes have been summarised and shown graphically in Fig. 2.2.

References

BARNETT, H. J. M., BOTTERELL, E. H., JOUSSE, A. T. and WYNN-JONES, MEGAN (1966) *Brain*, **89**, 159.

BORS, E. (1955) *Proceedings of the 4th Annual Clinical Spinal Cord Injury Conference*, p. 42. Washington: Amer. Vet. Adm.

CARAVATI, C., MOREY, D. A. J. and REGAN, W. W. (1958) *Gastroenterology*, **34**, 683.

DIETRICK, R. B. and RUSSI, S. (1958) *J. Amer. Med. Ass.*, **166**, 41.

GUTTMANN, L. (1953) *Medical History of the Second World War*; *Surgery*, pp. 422–516. Ed. Z. Cope. London: H.M.S.O.

GUTTMANN, L. (1962) *Monthly Bull. of Min. of Health and P.H.L.S.*, **21**, 60.

GUTTMANN, L. and SILVER, J. R. (1965) *Int. J. Paraplegia*, **3**, 1.

KAWAICHI, G. W. (1960) *Proceedings of the 9th Annual Clinical Spinal Cord Injury Conference*, p. 104. Washington: Amer. Veterans Adm.

MELZAK, J. (1966) *Int. J. Paraplegia*, **4**, 85.

SILVER, J. R. (1968) *Int. J. Paraplegia*, **5**, 226.

TRIBE, C. R. (1963a) *Int. J. Paraplegia*, **1**, 19.

TRIBE, C. R. (1963b) *Post-mortem Findings in Paraplegic Patients*. D.M. Thesis, Oxford.

WALSH, J. J. and TRIBE, C. R. (1965) *Int. J. Paraplegia*, **3**, 209. (Abstract of Paper.)

WOLMAN, L. (1965) *Int. J. Paraplegia*, **2**, 213.

3

Renal Failure in Chronic Paraplegia

This chapter amplifies the previous statistical analysis, describes the pathological processes causing renal failure in paraplegia, and gives illustrative case histories.

Definition

In this series, patients were considered to have died in renal failure if clinical and laboratory evidence of progressive renal disease during life was confirmed by post-mortem findings of severe renal damage. In almost every patient there was laboratory evidence of a rising blood urea level over many months, with a figure greater than 100 mg per cent during the last week of life.

Incidence

The incidence of renal failure varies according to the type of paraplegia. Table 3.1 shows how the incidence is represented in this series.

TABLE 3.1

Incidence of renal failure in chronic paraplegia

No of necropsies	Type of paraplegia	No of patients dying in renal failure	Incidence %
46	Acute	0	0
117	Chronic: Death related to paraplegia	86	73·5
57	Chronic: Death unrelated to paraplegia	3	5·3
Total 220	Acute and Chronic	89	40·5

Aetiology

Four main factors contribute, either singly or in combination, to renal failure in chronic paraplegia. These are pyelonephritis, amyloidosis, hypertension secondary to chronic renal disease, and calculosis. A study of pathological material enables the first three factors to be assessed (Table 3.2).

TABLE 3.2

Factors producing renal failure in chronic paraplegia

GROUPS A AND C: DEATH DUE TO RENAL FAILURE RELATED TO PARAPLEGIA

AETIOLOGICAL FACTORS	NO OF CASES
Pyelonephritis alone	17
Pyelonephritis and amyloidosis	24
Pyelonephritis and hypertension	16
Pyelonephritis, amyloidosis, and hypertension	14
Amyloidosis alone	2
Amyloidosis and hypertension	2
No kidney material available for histology	11
Total	86

Of the 75 patients from whom kidney tissue was available for histological study—

Pyelonephritis contributed to renal
failure in   71 (95%)

Amyloidosis contributed to renal failure
in   42 (56%)
Hypertension contributed to renal failure
in   32 (43%)

Calculosis is a common finding in chronic paraplegics and was more common in those patients who
died in renal failure (Table 3.3). The significance of
calculosis of the urinary tract is difficult to assess
since the post-mortem incidence of this disease does
not indicate the damage caused by calculi during life.
Lithotomies on different portions of the urinary
tract were also more common among patients who
died from diseases related to their paraplegia. Calculosis will be further discussed in Chapter 5.

TABLE 3.3
Calculosis in chronic paraplegia

	Patients who died in renal failure (89 cases)		Patients who did not die in renal failure (85 cases)	
Calculosis of the upper urinary tract detected during life	35	} 39 % with calculi	15	} 18 % with calculi
No calculi detected during life	54		70	

Comparison of the Findings in This Series with Modern Literature

Modern papers describe few necropsies on paraplegic patients, and this makes strict comparison
with the findings in this series impossible. A few
authors have studied sufficient post-mortem material
to compare the incidence and causes of renal failure
and their figures (Table 3.4) will be considered first.

TABLE 3.4
Renal failure in paraplegia (*modern literature*)

Authors	No. of post-mortems	Death due to renal failure	%
1. Reingold, 1953	25	Not stated	
	17 traumatic cases	6	35
2. Dietrick and Russi, 1958	58	11	20
3. Breithaupt *et al.*, 1961	40	20	50
4. Pearce *et al.*, 1964	35	18	51·6
5. Nyquist and Bors, 1967	258 deaths	85	32·9
	(99 post-mortems)		
(*a*) Guttmann, 1953 Stoke Mandeville Hospital 1945–53	26 Chronic, death related to paraplegia	20	74
(*b*) Tribe, 1963a, 1963b Stoke Mandeville Hospital 1945–62	150 Acute and Chronic	66	44
	122 Chronic	66	54
	84 Chronic, death related to paraplegia	64	76
(*c*) Present series Stoke Mandeville Hospital 1945–65	220 Acute and Chronic	89	40·5
	174 Chronic	89	51
	117 Chronic, death related to paraplegia	86	73·5

1. Reingold (1953) considered in detail the findings in only 17 of 25 necropsies on traumatic paraplegics. He stated that 6 died from causes directly related to paraplegia. They all died in uraemia, associated with chronic pyelonephritis and amyloidosis (3 cases), chronic pyelonephritis with calculi (2 cases) and chronic pyelonephritis with widespread arteriosclerosis (1 case). This pattern of renal disease is closely comparable to the findings in the present series.

2. In 1958, Dietrick and Russi published *A Tabulation and Review of the Autopsy Findings in Fifty-five Paraplegics*. These autopsies were performed in 1946–55, and 41 (75%) cases were of traumatic origin. Their list of primary pathological diagnoses is headed by 11 patients (20%) who died from renal disease. Of the 11, 6 had acute and chronic pyelonephritis, 4 renal amyloidosis and 1 had renal failure due to generalised tuberculosis. Of their patients, 90·2 per cent had some form of genito-urinary disease related to paraplegia and 64·7 per cent had post-mortem evidence of pyelo-nephritis. It is difficult at first glance to see why these authors had such a low incidence of renal failure. However, they made no attempt to differentiate between acute and chronic cases or deaths related and unrelated to paraplegia, and, if 5 patients who died from infectious hepatitis are excluded, the degree and type of renal disease in this series is comparable to our own.

In their summary, Dietrick and Russi end by saying that 'the incidence of renal disease as a fatal complication is apparently decreasing in paraplegia'. In 1963, Tribe found no evidence to support this statement. In the present series, with larger numbers available for study over a longer period, this important point was reassessed. Table 4.5 compares the incidence of renal failure in the periods 1945–55 (the same period as the cases seen by Dietrick and Russi), 1956–62 (Tribe, 1963a), and 1962–65 (additional cases).

TABLE 3.5
Incidence of renal failure

CHRONIC PARAPLEGIA—DEATH RELATED TO PARAPLEGIA
(GROUPS A AND C)

	1945–55	1956–62	1962–65
Deaths from renal failure	34	30	22
Deaths from other causes	8	12	11

These results, in one spinal centre, confirm the statement by Dietrick and Russi that there is a trend towards a lower incidence of renal failure in chronic paraplegia. This is probably related to the steady

improvement in the overall mortality rate in these patients.

3. Breithaupt *et al.* (1961) reviewed the causes of death in paraplegics at Toronto General Hospital and Sunnybrook Veterans Hospital, between 1945 and 1958. Of 94 deaths in traumatic paraplegics during this period, they estimated that 40 (42·5%) died in renal failure. Of the 40 that came to necropsy, 20 (50%) had died from renal failure. Unfortunately, no further pathological details are given, but these figures agree fairly closely with those in our series.

4. Pearce *et al.* (1964) reviewed 35 necropsies on cases of spinal cord injury from the Veterans Hospital, Richmond, Virginia. They found that 18 out of the 32 chronic paraplegics died from renal failure (51·6%). Chronic and acute renal failure was the underlying cause in 16, and, although amyloidosis was present in 17 patients, it was the primary cause of renal failure in only 2 of them.

5. In a recent paper, Nyquist and Bors (1967) analysed the mortality and survival in 1,851 patients with traumatic myelopathy who had been treated at the Spinal Cord Injury Service, Veterans Administration Hospital, Long Beach, California, between 1946 and 1965. The mortality rate was 258 (13·9%), and they considered that 172 deaths (67%) were related (based on the criteria laid down by Tribe, 1963a), 58 (22%) were unrelated to the injury, and 28 deaths (11%) were undetermined. The cause of death was verified by autopsy in only 99 cases (38%). Renal failure was considered to be the cause of death in 85 out of the total 258 deaths (32·9%), but the authors do not give the separate incidence in their related and unrelated groups. Nor are separate figures given for the findings in the cases coming to autopsy, so strict comparison with this important paper is not possible.

Other papers which give statistics of the incidence of renal failure in chronic paraplegia, but without post-mortem details, include the following—

A. Truebeger (1958) analysed five years' mortality figures in the Spinal Cord Injury Service of Kennedy Veterans Administration Hospital, between 1953 and 1957. He considered that 19 of the chronic paraplegics died from pyelonephritis, and included 9 cases of secondary amyloidosis in his list of additional diagnoses.

B. Nyquist (1960) reviewed the 184 deaths in 1,626 patients from the Veterans Administration Hospital, Long Beach, California, between 1946 and 1960. The paraplegia was of traumatic origin in 141, and 104 had died from causes connected with the spinal cord injury. In this group, the main causes of death were renal (52), pulmonary (18), suicide (14), secondary amyloidosis (13), liver disease (9), peritonitis (6), and haemorrhage (6). Fifty per cent of his cases, therefore, died of renal disease and this figure is comparable with the findings in this series.

C. Hoffman and Bunts (1962) analysed material from 43 deaths in 156 Second World War paraplegics. Of these, 17 had died of renal disease after an average survival time of eight years nine months. No indication is given concerning the total number of necropsies, but they stated that, '90 per cent of all deaths proven at post-mortem had pathological processes in the kidneys'.

D. Other papers, written since the Second World War, giving mortality rates in paraplegics with percentages of patients dying from renal failure include Damanski and Gibbon (1956)—64 per cent; Lord and Bunts (1956)—38 per cent; and Barber and Cross (1952)—64 per cent. Bunts (1959) reviewed the mortality statistics in the paraplegic, and quoted eight authors who found that the percentage of deaths due to urinary tract disease varied from 20–64 per cent.

On comparing the three sets of mortality statistics and incidence of renal failure available from the material at Stoke Mandeville Hospital (Table 3.4 (a), (b), and (c)), it is remarkable how constant the incidence of renal failure in chronic paraplegics has remained over twelve years. In the group of patients dying from causes related to their paralysis the incidence has been as follows—74 per cent in 1953, 76 per cent in 1962, and 73·5 per cent in 1965. Only serial, rather than cumulative analysis, (Table 3.5) suggests that the incidence of renal failure is falling.

The incidence of renal failure in the series of other authors appears to be about 50 per cent, and the difference between this and our own average (around 75%) is probably due to two factors. First, the larger number of cases in our series has allowed us to make important sub-divisions and, although we feel that the best group for accurate comparison is the chronic paraplegics dying from causes related to their paralysis, our figures for the incidence of renal failure among all chronic paraplegics (54% and 51%) are comparable with the findings of other authors. Second, apart from the papers of Dietrick and Russi (1958) and Pearce *et al.* (1964) based on only 55 and 35 post-mortems respectively, there are no papers with comparable pathological details. Mortality statistics without full histopathological investigations are notoriously unreliable.

An interesting anomaly shown in this comparison with modern literature is the much lower incidence of amyloidosis, and the virtual absence of deaths due to hypertension secondary to chronic renal disease in other series. This will be analysed and discussed in later chapters.

Enough evidence has been presented at this stage to show that renal failure in chronic paraplegia is usually due to several factors. Analysis of these pathological factors and judgement of the part played by each in the ultimate cause of death, can only be made by a critical review of the clinical history, radiological and laboratory investigations during life, and the ultimate post-mortem findings. Two illustrative case-histories are now presented. These have been chosen deliberately to show the complex nature of renal disease in many of these patients.

Case History I

G. H. (Case no. 143), aged fifty-one at the time of his death in November 1961, had sustained a traumatic paraplegia sixteen years previously (in July 1945) after a road traffic accident while serving in the Forces in Germany. This resulted in paralysis, incomplete below C.7 and complete below T.3. An initial suprapubic cystotomy was closed after six months. He was first admitted to Stoke Mandeville Hospital in August 1949 with severe pressure sores of both buttocks.

Chronological list of significant clinical details—

September 1949 Intravenous pyelogram showed normal bilateral secretion with a calculus in the left kidney. Left nephrolithotomy.

September 1955 His original pressure sores were virtually healed by early 1950, but a sinus persisted over the right ischium and this was now excised with an underlying focus of osteomyelitis. Intravenous pyelogram still normal.

September 1960 Clinical evidence of hypertension was first noted. The blood pressure was 140/100 and rose to 200/130 at time of death. The blood urea first became raised at this time and remained above 80 mg per cent until death when it was 245 mg per cent.

October 1960 The urea clearance was now below 10 per cent and remained low until death. Gross proteinuria was also present and the plasma albumin was 1·4 G per cent.

November 1960 A second left nephrolithotomy was performed following X-ray evidence of recurrent calculi.

January 1961	Investigation of haematemesis was followed by partial gastrectomy for removal of a benign tumour of stomach (hamartoma).
May 1961	Removal of calculi from bladder.
October 1961	Became deeply comatose for last month of life.

Note. There had been (*a*) persistent urinary infection with *Pseudomonas pyocyanea* since time of injury, and by *Klebsiella aerogenes* since 1957, and (*b*) during the last year of life multiple blood transfusions and a high protein diet were given to combat persistent renal anaemia and gross hypoproteinaemia.

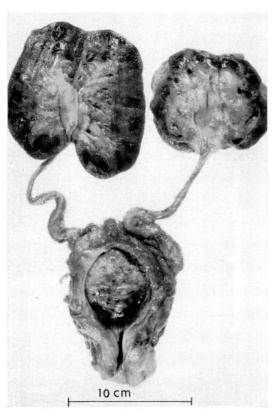

10 cm

Fɪɢ. 3.1. Urinary tract of G.H. Case History I described in the text.

RELEVANT POST-MORTEM FINDINGS

A massive haemorrhage into the left cerebral hemisphere was the major cause of death. The heart was enlarged (460 G) from left ventricular hypertrophy with only slight coronary atheroma. There were large pleural effusions and severe pulmonary oedema. The urinary tract is shown in Fig. 3.1, where the left

kidney can be seen to be grossly scarred with severe loss of renal tissue and a moderate hydronephrosis. The right kidney was normal in size and showed loss of cortico-medullary demarcation, and a generalised, firm, waxy pale blotchiness, characteristic of severe renal amyloidosis. The ureters were a little thickened and the bladder showed gross muscular hypertrophy of its wall with trabeculation and congestion of the mucosa.

On histological examination, the remaining tissue in the left kidney showed severe generalised chronic atrophic pyelonephritis with amyloid replacement of the few surviving glomeruli. In contrast, the right kidney showed only occasional small focal areas of chronic pyelonephritic scarring with gross amyloid infiltration of the glomeruli, peritubular regions and in the walls of the vessels. There was marked benign nephrosclerosis in both kidneys but no evidence of malignant hypertension (*see* Fig. 7.1). In addition, there was severe infiltration of the liver, spleen, and adrenals by amyloid material and this was demonstrated in small amounts in the tongue, thyroid, heart, pancreas, and rectum.

COMMENT

This case history clearly illustrates the complex nature of the pathological changes which develop as a direct result of the septic complications of chronic paraplegia. In this patient, chronic renal disease due to a combination of pyelonephritis, scarring following surgical removal of calculi and possibly amyloidosis led to severe secondary hypertension which eventually caused death by a massive cerebral haemorrhage.

The pressure sores and underlying osteomyelitis, although healed six years before death, were almost certainly the prime factor in the development of secondary amyloidosis which involved the kidneys to such a degree that death from renal failure was imminent before the cerebral haemorrhage occurred.

Case History II

N. H. (Case no. 202) aged forty-two at death in September 1964, had sustained a traumatic paraplegia from a gunshot wound twenty years previously (September 1944) with complete paralysis below L.2. Emergency treatment included a suprapubic cystotomy and laminectomy, and in 1947 calculi were removed from his bladder. He was first admitted to Stoke Mandeville Hospital in June 1948 with severe pressure sores of the sacrum and both buttocks, and chronic urinary infection.

Chronological list of significant clinical details—

| June 1948 | Epididymo-orchitis. |
| September 1950 | Suprapubic cystotomy closed after six years. |

1949, 1950, 1951 and 1952	Repeated operations for closure of chronic pressure sores including removal of osteomyelitic focus from the left ischium. No significant pressure sores since 1952.
1951	Calculus removed from bladder.
1952	Intravenous pyelogram showed moderate bilateral hydronephrosis.
October 1955	Intravenous pyelogram now normal.
December 1956	Intravenous pyelogram showed a small calculus in the left kidney. Left nephrolithotomy.
April 1960	The blood urea first became raised and remained above 50 mg per cent for the rest of his life.
June 1963	Urea clearance 22 per cent and 30 per cent and proteinuria 10·9 G every twenty-four hours.
October 1963	Severe hypertension with retinopathy. Previous blood pressure records, taken at least once a year since 1952, gave no warning of this rapid onset of malignant hypertension.
November 1963 until death	Blood pressure varied up to 230/140 despite treatment with Rauwiloid. Renal function gradually deteriorated with the blood urea reaching a terminal figure of 472 mg per cent. In July 1964, three months before death, the serum creatinine was 8·3 mg per cent and a creatinine clearance 3·9 ml/min. In the last few months of life he developed gross peripheral oedema and bilateral pleural effusions.

Note. At no time since the onset of paraplegia was the urine free from infection. Pathogenic organisms included *Ps. pyocyanea*, *E. coli*, *Proteus*, and *K. aerogenes*.

RELEVANT POST-MORTEM FINDINGS

There were bilateral pleural effusions with a chronic haemorrhagic fibrinous pericarditis. The heart was enlarged (570 G) from left ventricular hypertrophy, and the coronary arteries showed moderate atheroma. The lungs showed gross pulmonary oedema and basal collapse. The kidneys were equally reduced in size (200 G combined weight), and there was perinephric fibrosis and scarring at the upper pole of the left kidney and in the midzone of the right kidney. Small recent petechial haemorrhages were present beneath the capsules, suggestive of the 'flea-bitten' appearance of malignant hypertension. On section, there was a mild bilateral hydronephrosis and blurring of the cortico-medullary margins. The renal cortex had a firm, white waxiness suggestive of amyloidosis.

On histological examination, there were focal areas of atrophic chronic pyelonephritis in the upper pole of the left kidney and amyloid material had virtually replaced all the glomerular tufts. There was marked endarteritis and intimal proliferation of the smaller renal arteries and approximately 5 per cent of the glomeruli showed 'crescent' formation confirming malignant nephrosclerosis. Amyloid infiltration was moderate in the spleen, and small amounts were detected in the thyroid, liver, adrenals, pancreas, tongue, stomach, duodenum, lymph nodes, prostate, bone-marrow, choroid plexus, and pituitary.

COMMENT

This case history also shows a complex pathological picture and illustrates several points—

1. The late development of severe hypertension which was of malignant type as soon as it was noted.
2. The hypertension which was almost certainly secondary, and was probably due to scarring of the kidneys from focal chronic pyelonephritis and surgical removal of renal calculi.
3. The renal failure which was predominantly due to amyloidosis and malignant nephrosclerosis.
4. The long interval between apparent removal and cure of the chief aetiological agents (pressure sores and osteomyelitis), and clinical evidence of amyloidosis.

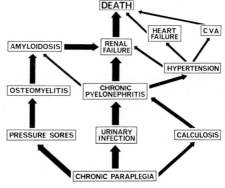

FIG. 3.2

In analysis of the original 150 post-mortem cases, the author made a diagram showing the way in which the pathological processes resulting from the septic complications of chronic paraplegia led to death (Tribe, 1963a, 1963b) and it is considered worthwhile reproducing it (Fig. 3.2).

Although each individual case follows a different pathway, with differing accents on the various stages, Fig. 3.2 shows the predominant part played by renal failure in the cause of death in chronic paraplegics, and also illustrates its mixed aetiology.

References

BARBER, K. E. and CROSS, R. R. (1952) *J. Urol.*, **67**, 494.

BREITHAUPT, D. J., JOUSSE, A. T. and WYNN-JONES, M. (1961) *Canad. Med. Ass. J.*, **85**, 73.

BUNTS, R. C. (1959) *J. Urol.*, **81**, 720.

DAMANSKI, M. and GIBBON, N. (1956) *Brit. J. Urol.*, **28**, 24.

DIETRICK, R. B. and RUSSI, S. (1958) *J. Amer. Med. Ass.*, **166**, 41.

GUTTMANN, L. (1953) *Medical History of the Second World War. Surgery*, pp. 422–515. Ed. Z. Cope. London: H.M.S.O.

HOFFMAN, C. A. and BUNTS, R. C. (1962) *J. Urol.*, **86**, 60.

LORD, K. H. and BUNTS, R. C. (1956) *J. Urol.*, **75**, 66.

NYQUIST, R. H. (1960) *Proceedings of the 9th Annual Clinical Spinal Cord Injury Conference*, p. 109. Amer. Veterans Adm.

NYQUIST, R. H. and BORS, E. (1967) *Int. J. Paraplegia*, **5**, 22.

PEARCE, L. S., PERKINS, H. E. and HOLLADAY, L. W. (1964) *Proceedings of the 13th Annual Clinical Spinal Cord Injury Conference*, p. 88. Amer. Veterans Adm.

REINGOLD, I. M. (1953) *Proceedings of the 2nd Annual Clinical Spinal Cord Injury Conference*, p. 1. Amer. Veterans Adm.

TRIBE, C. R. (1963a) *Int. J. Paraplegia*, **1**, 19.

TRIBE, C. R. (1963b) *Post-mortem Findings in Paraplegic Patients*. D.M. Thesis. Oxford.

TRUEBEGER, H. M. (1958) *Proceedings of the 7th Annual Clinical Spinal Cord Injury Conference*, p. 164. Amer. Veterans Adm.

4
Diagnostic Tests for Urinary Tract Disease in Chronic Paraplegia

<hr>

IF A PARAPLEGIC patient survives the first three months after injury, his life expectancy is almost entirely determined by the functional integrity of his kidneys. Much of the renal damage is caused by incomplete emptying of the bladder, which leads to stasis, infection, and back pressure effects on the kidney.

The urine of chronic paraplegics must be examined frequently for infection, and repetitive tests of bladder and renal function are necessary to diagnose renal damage in its early stages so that appropriate treatment can be started. In the later stages of renal disease these tests also have prognostic value.

Since paralysis of the bladder is the key to the sequence of events leading to renal failure in paraplegia, the physiology of normal micturition and its alteration by spinal cord disease will be considered first.

The Physiology of Micturition

Micturition depends on a spinal reflex mediated by the mid-sacral segments but under the higher control of the mid-brain, thalamus, subcortical centres, and frontal lobes of the brain. The bladder is innervated from three main sources, the parasympathetic which constitutes the motor efferent supply from the mid-sacral segments, the sympathetic via the hypogastric nerves which supply the trigone, and the voluntary nerve supply to the external sphincter and pelvic floor from the pudendal nerves.

The bladder is a fibro-muscular organ mainly composed of smooth muscle, but at its floor, enclosing the internal urethral orifice, there is a reinforcement of collagenous connective tissue, the so-called baseplate (Hutch, 1966). In addition, voluntary muscle is present within the urethra as high as the internal urinary orifice (the so-called internal sphincter), where it blends with the smooth muscle of the bladder. This voluntary muscle produces increased resistance to the passage of urine in the urethra 2–3 cm distal to the prostate, where the urethra passes through the pelvic diaphragm (the external sphincter) (Ross et al., 1957, 1963; Smythe 1966). The ureters enter the bladder obliquely at the trigone, and their obliquity and healthy mucosa prevent urine from refluxing up the ureters. Normally, the bladder stores urine at low pressure, and the urethra can withstand pressures of up to 30–50 cm of water without opening. The gradual filling of the bladder by urine initiates small reflex contractions of the detrusor which may be suppressed or reinforced by the higher centres. When bladder pressure is raised by coughing, straining, or voluntary effort mediated by the parasympathetic nerves, a strong contraction of the whole detrusor complex of the bladder follows, the base plate of the bladder descends, and the internal urethral orifice is taken up and is pulled open as part of the contraction. There is a reciprocal relaxation of the pelvic floor, and with it the external sphincter, and micturition occurs. The role of the external sphincter is critical. At rest this muscle does not contract but if a normal subject coughs, strains, stands, or finds it inconvenient to micturate for social reasons, the external sphincter contracts vigorously and can retain the urine within the bladder, although this can be a painful process (Susset et al., 1965).

Effects on the Bladder Following Spinal Transection

The disturbances of micturition that follow spinal injury depend upon the anatomical level of the injury and upon the length of time since injury. The complicating influence of infection will be discussed later.

ANATOMICAL LEVEL

Two patterns of disturbance of micturition can be distinguished, depending upon the anatomical level: (Gibbon, 1966).

1. If the lower motor neurone arc controlling the bladder is interrupted on either the motor or sensory side by damage to the spinal cord or the mid-sacral nerves in their pathway through the pelvis, the reflex pathways controlling micturition are interrupted, this causes a lower motor neurone paralysis of the bladder and reflex detrusor contractions cannot take place.
2. If the lesion is above the sacral segments and the lower motor neurone arc is preserved, an upper motor neurone paralysis occurs and an uninhibited reflex detrusor contraction may take place (free of descending inhibition or reinforcement from the higher centres).

LENGTH OF TIME AFTER SPINAL INJURY

1. *Lower motor neurone bladder in the stage of spinal shock.* Damage to the sacral segments interrupts the reflex pathways for micturition and this can be demonstrated by the absence of the anal and bulbo cavernosus reflexes. There is a total retention of urine due to the natural closed state of the urethra. This retention is independent of nervous impulses since it persists at post-mortem (Gibbon, 1950), and in the presence of pudendal nerve block and muscular paralysis produced by relaxants (Lapides *et al.*, 1957). In all these conditions, the bladder has been found to be full of urine although suprapubic pressure can expel it. The abdominal muscles, if they are above the level of injury, retain their power. Sensation from the bladder may still be appreciated via the sympathetic nerves.
2. *Lower motor neurone bladder when spinal shock has subsided.* When the stage of spinal shock has subsided, reflex activity of the bladder will still be absent since the reflex arc has been interrupted. Emptying of the bladder will depend upon abdominal straining or manual compression. Sensation of bladder distension may still be preserved, via the sympathetic nerves. These patients frequently complain of incontinence due to distension of the bladder with overflow. This may take place even when there is only a small quantity of urine in the bladder, owing to the flaccidity and paralysis of the pelvic floor and external sphincter.
3. *Upper motor neurone bladder in the stage of spinal shock.* If the lesion is above the sacral segments, the reflex pathways for micturition are still intact. This can be demonstrated by the preservation of the anal and bulbo cavernosus reflexes immediately after cord injury. In the stage of spinal shock, the reflex contractions of the bladder are depressed, but they may return as quickly as seventy-two hours after injury in a young patient,

although they may not be powerful enough to take up the internal sphincter and ensue complete emptying of the bladder. There will be retention of urine due to the natural closed state of the urethra.
4. *Upper motor neurone bladder when spinal shock has subsided.* When the stage of spinal shock has subsided in patients with lesions above the sacral segments, spinal reflex micturition is possible. The bladder is stimulated to contract by the presence of quite small quantities of urine. This is in contrast to a normal subject in whom these reflex contractions are suppressed until it is convenient to micturate. Incontinence may result from this, and from the inco-ordinated contraction of the bladder, the pelvic floor, and the adductors of the thigh. Normally, the pelvic floor and the adductor muscles relax during micturition, but in a patient with marked spasticity micturition is often interrupted by a flexor spasm in which the external sphincter closes the urethra so that incomplete emptying of the bladder results. The patient complains of dribbling and spurts of urine.

EFFECTS OF URINARY INFECTION

During the stage of spinal shock the bladder must be drained, since in all lesions, apart from the very incomplete ones, the detrusor contractions are not powerful enough to empty the bladder. It is at this stage that infection is introduced, and there is clear evidence that the mode of introduction of infection is by the catheter. During the First World War 80 per cent of paraplegic patients died from ascending urinary infection (Thompson Walker, 1917). When special precautions are taken by using a non-touch technique with intermittent catheterisation (Frankel and Guttmann, 1965), or when the urethra is irrigated with antiseptic solution and a special light weight catheter is left *in situ* (Gibbon 1958; MacLeod *et al.*, 1963), the urine may be kept sterile for several weeks. The skill with which the catheterisation is performed is critical, and if these precautions are not taken then infection of the bladder occurs within forty-eight hours.

However, the introduction of bacteria by a catheter into a normal bladder is not sufficient to result in permanent urinary infection. This has been shown by Cattell *et al.* (1963) when he followed 102 non-paraplegic female patients who had developed a bladder infection after a vaginal repair in 1953. Nine years later, no patient was found to have progressive renal damage that could be attributed to their catheter induced infection of 1953. Lepper (1921) and Heptinstall and Brumfitt (1960) have shown that pyelonephritis occurs when there is some anatomical abnormality present which causes obstruction, in addition to the presence of pathogenic organisms. This has been emphasised by the observation of Schoenberg *et al.* (1964), who found that it was impossible to produce chronic lower urinary tract infection in animals without traumatising the bladder as well as introducing infection.

The normal bladder has self-sterilising mechanisms, the most important of which is complete emptying, so that even if pathogenic organisms are introduced into the cavity of the bladder, it remains free of infection. In the paraplegic patient, where this mechanism is impaired and incomplete emptying results, the bladder becomes rapidly infected following introduction of pathogenic organisms. When this infection becomes established, it spreads from within the cavity of the bladder to the bladder wall, causing fibrosis of the bladder neck so that it becomes rigid and no longer taken up by the detrusor contraction of the bladder. The fibrosis and oedema spread to involve the ureteric orifices so that they became patulous, and infected urine is free to regurgitate up the ureter to the kidney giving rise to pyelonephritis, hydronephrosis, and destruction of the kidney.

THE INFLUENCE OF PRESSURES WITHIN THE BLADDER

In the initial stages immediately after spinal cord transection, when there is no reflex activity present within the bladder, the bladder must be drained to prevent permanent damage to its wall by over-distension (Bors, 1957; Cook, 1960; Band, 1961). Whether, or not, keeping the bladder permanently empty by the use of an indwelling catheter delays the return of reflex activity is controversial. Munro (1936) believed that regular distension of the bladder facilitates a return of reflex activity. He achieved this by the use of tidal drainage equipment. Guttmann (Frankel and Guttmann, 1965) achieved the same effect by means of intermittent catheterisation, allowing the bladder to distend regularly in the initial stages after cord injury. Guttmann's practice is followed at the Liverpool Regional Paraplegic Centre, where all new traumatic cases are treated by intermittent catheterisation unless there is severe infection of the urinary tract. During the last two years, 12 patients have been treated in this way: 10 achieved a satisfactory pattern of micturition between ten days and nine weeks after paralysis, with negligible sterile residual urines and normal upper renal tracts as shown by intravenous pyelography. Similar results have been achieved in Poland (Gibbon, personal communication), although Bors (1966), Hardy (1966), and Damanski (1967) have not found the method satisfactory.

Theoretical support for the clinical observations of Munro and Guttmann have been afforded by the animal experiments of Bradley *et al.* (1963), who showed that the detrusor becomes inefficient when left undistended for several weeks. The long-term effects of permanent catheter drainage have been analysed by Pritzl and Bors (1966). The patients without catheters had larger bladders than those with catheters. Considerable pressures may be achieved within the bladder, reflexly or by straining. If there is free drainage of urine, there will be no permanent changes to the bladder or ureters. However, if there is obstruction, the most common causes of which are fibrosis of the bladder neck due to infection, stones within the bladder, an enlarged prostate, or skeletal spasm involving the pelvic floor and adductor muscles, then the bladder becomes hypertrophied, fibrotic and trabeculated. The ureteric orifices become patulous and patent, and the raised pressures within the bladder are transmitted to the kidneys. This results in hydronephrosis, and the increased intra-renal pressure results in a fall in renal blood flow. The secretion of urine is gradually diminished and there are concomitant changes in renal metabolism. Schirmer *et al.* (1966) have shown experimentally in dogs that when the ureter is occluded there is a decrease in oxidative metabolism and an increase in anaerobic metabolism.

If the obstruction to the urine outflow is eliminated early, the bladder will regain its normal structure and function. If the obstruction is long continued, the bladder becomes permanently fibrotic and unable to contract, and acute pyelonephritis develops from the ascent of infected urine that is injected with considerable force into the substance of the kidney when the urine outflow is obstructed (Hodson, 1967). When this obstruction is relieved, the kidney may regain its normal function. However, 'the changes produced in the renal parenchyma and pelves by sufficiently severe or recurrent infections may themselves perpetuate the tendency to infection and the development of chronic pyelonephritis' (De Wardener, 1967).

Prolonged infection causes fibrosis, and even before permanent structural changes take place, it causes an alteration in the excitability of the bladder, increasing the pressures generated within. Sommer and Roberts (1966) showed that when *Proteus* infection was present in the bladders of a group of dogs much higher pressures were generated, and there was a much higher incidence of ureteric reflux than in a control group free of infection. It is a frequent observation that when a new traumatic paraplegic has been successfully treated by intermittent catheterisation, a severe infection develops just when automatic micturition begins to be established and the patient starts to expel urine spontaneously. The explanation is presumably that the infection stimulates the bladder to contract more forcibly.

It can thus be seen how, after damage to the spinal cord, infection and the altered pressures developed within the bladder interact to damage the kidneys. Once this damage has been initiated, pyelonephritis, stones, and amyloidosis, and eventually hypertension, will supervene to complete the destruction of the kidneys.

Bacteriology

It is apparent from the other chapters in this monograph, that the success with which urinary tract infection is controlled directly affects the life expectancy of the paraplegic patient. Unlike normal medical practice where the physician looks for renal infection, often in the presence of sterile urine, as a cause of hypertension, proteinuria, or anaemia, the doctor concerned with paraplegic patients is faced usually with a plethora of infection and his problems are then therapeutic rather than diagnostic. Sometimes infection is found in a specimen of 'clean urine' and the problem then is whether this indicates contamination or infection of the urethra, bladder, or kidneys. Here, routine bacteriology must be supplemented by quantitative bacterial counts (*Lancet*, 1964), urinary white cell excretion rates (Hutt *et al.*, 1961), and pyrogen and prednisolone stimulation tests (De Wardener, 1967).

It has not been found necessary or desirable at the Liverpool Regional Paraplegic Centre to pass ureteric catheters to obtain specimens of urine from the kidney, because of the danger of introducing infection from the bladder to the kidneys. Morales (1967) obtained urine samples from the bladders and kidneys of 10 paraplegics at cystoscopy. Of these, 3 patients had infected kidney and bladder samples, 5 had only infected bladder samples, and in 2 patients all the samples were sterile. He concluded that, in paraplegics, the kidneys may remain uninfected in the presence of marked bladder infection, but that, in time, the infection would spread from the bladder to the kidneys.

In controlling urinary infection in paraplegic patients, the practice at Stoke Mandeville should be followed. The doctor takes all specimens of urine through a freshly passed catheter with full aseptic precautions and takes the specimen immediately to the laboratory. With out-patients, careful mid-stream specimens are taken and examined as soon as possible. In the laboratory, the urine samples are cultured and cell counts and examination of the urinary deposits undertaken. A special serial card of

all urinary infections in each paraplegic patient is kept in the laboratory with a duplicate copy in the clinical notes. Each day, the clinician and the pathologist inspect the cultures and sub-cultures (as detailed by Milner in 1963) and, thus, a close watch on all urinary infections and their response to treatment can be maintained. In addition, a chart of all urinary infections (with different coloured pins for different organisms) in the paraplegic wards is kept up to date to watch for cross-infection. Close co-operation between the clinicians, bacteriologist, and laboratory technicians is the keystone to this system.

There are many problems concerning the natural history of urinary tract infections in paraplegics, and the response to treatment, that require further research—

1. What part is played by organisms from the patient's own gastro-intestinal tract in causing bladder infection? Are they the normal source of infection of the bladder, or do the organisms come from other patients under treatment in the Centre?
2. After effective treatment of a urinary infection what does reappearance of the same organism at a later date indicate? Does it indicate recrudescence of the organism, or is it a fresh infection?
3. What is the correct duration of antibiotic treatment for different types of pathogens?
4. What part can long-term chemotherapy play?

Brumfitt and Percival (1963) have shown that problems of this kind can be solved by meticulous bacteriology and typing of organisms, and correlation with antibody studies.

Assessment of Residual Urine

The residual urine is the amount left within the bladder after the act of micturition, and is normally nil. If an infection develops in the bladder of a normal person, then all the infected urine will be passed each time the patient micturates. This is an important self-sterilising mechanism. In contrast, if a patient with an anatomical abnormality, such as an enlarged prostate or a paralysed bladder (which gives rise to residual urine), develops a urinary infection there will be a persistent residuum of infection within the bladder. This residual urine serves as a focus to infect fresh urine secreted by the kidneys. O'Grady and Cattell (1966) have demonstrated that the rate of multiplication of bacteria within the bladder is logarythmic and is reduced by two factors, the frequency of bladder emptying and the size of the residual urine. O'Grady and Pennington (1967) have shown that the concentration of the bacteria, as opposed to their rate of multiplication, is affected by the quantity of urine secreted by the kidneys into the bladder, since a large quantity of fresh urine will dilute the culture within the bladder. They also showed that the resistance of bacteria within the bladder to antibiotics is modified by their concentration, so that a severe bladder infection with a high concentration of bacteria requires much larger quantities of antibiotics to inhibit growth than a more dilute urine. These theoretical concepts support the practical advice that is given to paraplegic patients to empty their bladders regularly by the clock at hourly intervals. When a patient develops a severe urinary infection, his residual urine must be reduced to nil by an indwelling catheter, and the concentration of bacteria within the bladder reduced by giving plenty of fluids.

It naturally follows that the assessment of the residual urine is of considerable importance. It is essential to ensure that the patient empties his bladder under optimal conditions. This is best ensured by the doctor himself performing the residual check and determining first that the patient uses whatever tricks he has learnt, such as tapping on the abdomen or straining at the toilet, to empty his bladder. One source of error has been demonstrated by Cook (1960) who showed that, in the recumbent position, urine pools at the back of the bladder and despite washing through an indwelling Foley catheter all the urine is not obtained. Once the patient is sat up, however, further urine can be drained. These findings were confirmed by Doggart *et al.* (1966) who carried out similar studies on 20 paraplegic patients and found that when the patient stood up, after a conventional residual check, as much as 16 ml more urine could be obtained.

The significance of the residual urine must be assessed. A record of its quantity, and whether it is infected or sterile, is not the only information required. Some patients who were heavy beer drinkers before their paraplegia, may have been in the habit of suppressing the desire to micturate and may have bladders with capacities of up to 2 pints. In these people, the finding of a sterile residual urine of 3–4 oz may be acceptable. On the other hand, in a patient who has a small contracted fibrotic bladder with a total capacity of only 2 oz, the urine may be all residual and if infected is of much greater significance. Bors (1957) attempted to relate these factors by determining a ratio (expressed as a percentage) between the residual urine and the total bladder capacity, based on a minimum bladder capacity of 250 cm³. He found residual urines of up to 20 per cent in cases with upper, and 10 per cent in those with lower, motor neurone lesions were empirically compatible with satisfactory bladder function. The danger of his reasoning is that infection itself affects the bladder emptying, and it is the total quantity of infected urine left in the bladder that affects the rate of multiplication of bacteria, not the relationship of the residual urine to the total capacity of the bladder. Probably the most satisfactory definition of an acceptable residual urine is the one made by Gibbon (1966) who defines it as one that 'will remain sterile, and leaves the upper urinary tracts free from dilatation'.

Assessment of Bladder Pressures

Cystometry is a controversial method of investigating bladder function. 'It discloses the general condition of the neuromuscular detrusor unit, tone and adjustability to volume responsiveness to stretch and proprioception', i.e. desire to void and pain (Bors, 1957). The earliest estimations of bladder pressures in humans were made by Dubois (1876), but the whole subject was placed on a scientific basis by Rose (1927) and Denny-Brown and Robertson (1933a, 1933b). Controversy centres mainly around its value as a diagnostic procedure. The proponent Rose (1927) claimed that it yields information unobtainable from other sources, and the sceptics, Gibbon (1950) and Bors (1957), feel that cystometry is only one of many diagnostic tools and does not provide the diagnosis *per se*. The other less controversial, but more confusing, point is its use in classifying disorders of micturition. Here, the argument is largely one of semantics, as different terms are used by different authors to describe their findings. The experimental procedure employed at the Liverpool Regional Paraplegic Centre will first be described, the terms defined, and the value of cystometry discussed.

TECHNIQUE

Various forms of apparatus have been devised. At the Liverpool Regional Paraplegic Centre, the patient is examined supine, a soft rubber catheter of 18–20 Charier is used and the bladder is filled with sterile saline solution from an intravenous infusion bottle by means of an intravenous giving set. A T sidearm is connected through a tambour and the pressures are recorded on an aneroid manometer (Yeates, 1954). After 50 ml of saline have entered the bladder the reflex contractions are observed. The patient is asked to cough, take a deep breath, strain, sit up, and strain again, so that the maximum pressure generated within the bladder can be assessed. The procedure is repeated at 100, 200, 300, and 400 ml. The pulse, blood pressure, and any subjective sensations are recorded and the presence of sweating noted. This is of particular importance in lesions above T.5, where autonomic hyperreflexia is present.

This technique, whereby the bladder is rapidly filled, has been criticised by Comarr (1956). He points out that rapid filling of the bladder serves as a very strong stimulus to the bladder wall and that stronger contractions than normal will be obtained at a smaller volume. He recommends excretory cystometry, whereby the bladder is allowed to fill normally by urine and then the pressures recorded.

A NORMAL CYSTOMETROGRAM

With a slow continuous inflow, the intravesical pressure rises at first only very gradually, the bladder relaxing to store urine at a low pressure. When the limit of capacity is approached, pressure rises more quickly. The limit of capacity is taken as the point where involuntary emptying occurs and this ranges from about 200–800 ml, depending on the rate of flow.

In patients with spinal cord disease variations from the normal are seen—

Reflex Contractions

These are dependent on intact pathways from the bladder to the spinal cord and back to the bladder. Their characteristics are slow development, sustained high pressure, often accompanied by leakage around the catheter, and slow regression. They are independent of respiration, and each may consist of several small contractions fused together. The catheter may be rejected during a contraction, as the pressure developed may exceed 100–200 ml water.

Illustrative Case

J. P. had a motor cycle accident in 1963, resulting in a complete spastic lesion below T.5. He was discharged home, but his residual urine was found to be 6 oz in 1967. He stated that when he coughed, a stream of urine came out quite easily, but when he strained micturition was often stopped by a spasm of his legs. The cystometrogram showed that he had powerful contractions at volumes of 150 and 200 ml. The intravesical pressure rose to over 60 cm of water and forced out urine around the catheter. (*See* Fig. 4.1 III.)

Intravesicular Pressure

This is the pressure recorded from the bladder at any point of filling. It rises gradually as fluid enters the bladder until the limit of capacity is reached. It is largely dependent upon the condition of the intrinsic ganglia of the bladder wall, and has been shown to remain during spinal shock and cauda equina lesions, spinal anaesthesia, subarachnoid alcohol block, and pharmacological ganglionic paralysis (McLellan *et*

al., 1939; Nesbit, 1948; Sheldon and Bors, 1948; Boyce *et al.*, 1953), provided that the bladder is not overdistended. Gibbon (1950) found that in 12 normal subjects the pressure ranged from 1–11 cm of water in an empty bladder to 3–19 cm of water with 350 ml of water in the bladder.

Illustrative Case

This is well borne out by the pressure curves in E. J. (Fig. 4.1 I). After laminectomy (20/6/67) for a prolapsed thoracic intravertebral disc, this patient's lower limbs were flaccid and the tendon reflexes absent. A cystometrogram was carried out on 3 July 1967. There was complete absence of reflex contraction of the bladder but the intravesical pressure rose progressively as saline was added to the bladder. Straining or coughing raised the pressure. However, when the tendon reflexes later returned to his lower limbs and spasticity had developed, powerful detrusor contractions were present. On the cystometrogram (Fig. 4.1 II), which was repeated on 30 November 1967, it can be seen that the total capacity of the bladder is much smaller although the pressure is the same as before.

Maximum Voiding Pressures

These show a rapid rise, but are only maintained while respiration is arrested. On resumption of breathing, the pressure falls abruptly. They are almost certainly due to the transmission of pressures from the abdominal cavity to the bladder. This is particularly important in patients with no reflex contractions, as in tabes dorsalis or a severe cauda equina lesion. In these patients, the abdominal muscles are powerful and the patient can empty his bladder satisfactorily if he is instructed to strain.

Illustrative Case

1. P. S. had a cauda equina lesion after a fracture-dislocation of his 12th thoracic vertebra in 1961. He had normal abdominal muscles but anaesthesia and paralysis in the sacral segments. The anal reflex was absent. The cystometrogram showed that there were no reflex contractions, but there were very powerful maximum voiding pressures up to 200 cm of water, quite sufficient to empty his bladder (Fig. 4.1 V).

2. A similar picture is shown by R. P. who had tabes dorsalis for many years (Fig. 4.1 VI). His distended bladder was probably secondary to the absence of sensation of bladder distension. He had no reflex contractions, little sensation in the bladder apart from burning at 100 ml, but very powerful voiding pressures.

The Hypo-active Bladder

There are no reflex voiding contractions. This occurs when there is injury to the reflex from the bladder to the spinal cord and back to the bladder.

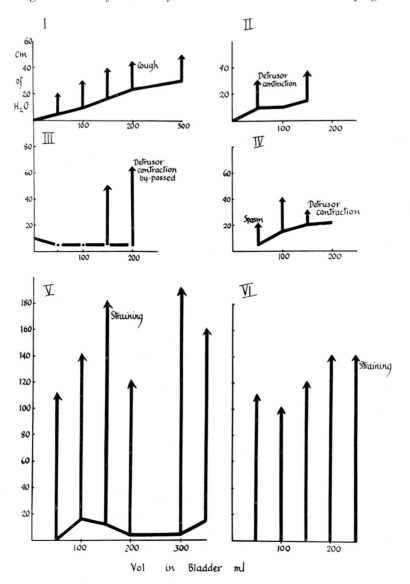

FIG. 4.1. Assessment of bladder pressures by cystometry.

I. E. J. in a state of spinal shock. No detrusor contractions. Normal basic tone. Anal reflex present.

II. E. J. five months later. Spasticity present in his lower limbs. Powerful detrusor contractions.

III. J. P. Powerful detrusor contractions. By-passing the catheter.

IV. M. W. Tetraplegic patient with weak detrusor contractions associated with autonomic hyperreflexia.

V. P. S. Cauda equina lesion. High voiding pressures. No detrusor contractions associated with patulous anus and absent anal and bulbocavernous reflexes. Note the difference between this patient with the absent anal reflex and the preceding cases where it was present (I–IV).

VI. R. P. with tabes dorsalis and absent tendon reflexes. High painful voiding contractions. No detrusor contractions.

The Hyper-active Bladder

There is a lowered threshold to the stretch reflex. The reflex pathways from the bladder to the spinal cord and back to the bladder are intact, but there is damage above the spinal cord. The voiding contractions are exaggerated and may be elicited by smaller stimuli. As little as 50–150 ml of urine in the bladder may precipitate these contractions. In some of the cervical and upper thoracic injuries they may produce autonomic hyperreflexia.

Illustrative Case

M. W. sustained a severe head injury on 12 December 1966, resulting in total paralysis below C.6. Anal reflex present. Cystometrogram, 5 July 1967, shows weak detrusor contractions associated with autonomic hyper-reflexia during which his blood pressure rose from 160/90 before cystometry to 205/120 with 200 ml of saline in the bladder (Fig. 4.1 IV).

CLINICAL VALUE

From the foregoing it should be stressed that the cystometrogram is not used to establish the diagnosis, but as a guide to treatment. Power, sensation and reflexes return at different rates to the striped voluntary muscles of the limbs and the skin overlying them, compared with the smooth muscle of the bladder. Thus, it is not uncommon to see satisfactory reflex emptying of the bladder occurring in a young patient within 2–3 weeks of a complete transection of the cord, if the urine is kept sterile, but no return of power to his lower limbs. On the other hand, when severe infection occurs and the bladder is damaged by overdistension the reflexes may return to the limbs, but the bladder remains atonic for a considerable period. The determination of the reflex contractions of the bladder and the maximum pressures that a patient can achieve by straining, sitting up, or compressing the bladder with the hands, is an excellent guide to the ultimate functional capability of the bladder. If a patient can achieve a pressure in his bladder of 30–40 cm water then it is worthwhile carrying out several bladder neck and external sphincter divisions to make the passage of urine easy, so that the patient can achieve satisfactory micturition. However, in many of the tetraplegic patients (Silver and Gibbon, 1968) where the emptying pressures are small, it may be necessary to accept that an indwelling catheter is the treatment of choice.

Radiological Investigations

Most of the information about the long-term effects of injuries to the spinal cord upon renal and bladder function has been obtained by radiological means. Many papers correlate the renal appearance, as shown radiologically, with the prognosis of the patient (Talbot and Bunts, 1949; Comarr 1954; Lord and Bunts, 1956; Damanski and Gibbon, 1956; Guttmann, 1963; Cobb and Talbot, 1966; Nyquist and Bors, 1967).

Two procedures are commonly used, intravenous pyelography and cystourethrography. Retrograde pyelography is seldom used because of the dangers of introducing infected urine from the bladder into the kidneys, and because modern excretion pyelography gives just as much information. Aortography is similarly not used since its value is in the investigation of patients with hypertension, to determine whether it is due to a remediable unilateral arterial anomaly. As has been explained earlier, renal disease in paraplegic patients is secondary to the ascent of infected urine from the bladder and, as such, is usually bilateral.

INTRAVENOUS PYELOGRAPHY

Intravenous pyelography tests two different aspects of renal function, glomerular filtration and, to a lesser degree, tubular secretion. It has many uses including the demonstration of stones, hydronephrosis, and chronic back pressure, shrinkage of the kidney from pyelonephritis, ureteric reflux, obstruction of the lower urinary tract, and, by means of a post micturition film, assessment of the residual urine without the passage of a catheter. The standard use of the technique enables results of tests carried out at different Centres to be compared. The fact that the films are seen independently by a Radiologist as well as the Clinician responsible for the management of the patient, introduces a degree of objectivity.

Technique (Double dose procedure)

Careful preparation of the patient to eliminate gas and faeces is necessary, and, for this reason, patients are admitted overnight and given a suppository. Improved concentration of the media is achieved by dehydrating the patient overnight, and in order to obtain satisfactory filling of the calyces a catheter, if present, is removed. At the Liverpool Regional Paraplegic Centre 40–50 ml of 60 per cent contrast medium are given as a standard procedure. Films are taken at 2, 5, 15 and 30 min. Bladder and oblique films are taken at 45 min. If the patient can micturate, a post micturition film is taken to assess the residual urine. A compression band is applied to the ureters, to retain the dye in the calyceal system of the kidneys.

If adequate visualisation is not obtained by this double dose procedure, *infusion pyelography* is carried out. A rapid intravenous infusion of 250 ml of 25 per cent contrast medium is given. Films are taken at 2, 5, 10, 15, and 30 min. A bladder film is also taken at 45 min. The infusion technique has several advantages. Conditions are more physiological as there is no need to dehydrate the patient, and no compression is applied. Since no overnight preparation is necessary, it is useful in abdominal emergencies in paraplegic patients, to investigate an impacted stone in the ureter or a suspected pyonephrosis. It gives better pictures showing the whole thickness of the kidney in the early filling phase (nephrogram) so that shrinkage can be determined, and it sometimes gives satisfactory pictures in the presence of renal impairment, when no picture is obtainable by the conventional double dose technique. An intravenous pyelogram may be supplemented by tomographs to give further information about the renal thickness and the localisation of a renal stone. The specific value of intravenous pyelography is in the diagnosis of—

1. *Hydronephrosis.* In its early stages, this cannot be detected by other means.

2. *Ureteric reflux.* Cobb and Talbot (1966) have shown that there is a fullness of the lower ureters in the conventional pyelogram which correlates with the cystographic finding of reflux.

3. *Renal stones.* The combination of tomography and infusion pyelography is valuable in showing in which calyx a stone is situated.

4. *Chronic pyelonephritis.* Hodson (1959) has pointed out that scarring, which is a radiological sign of pyelonephritis, only occurs in children when there

is active regrowth of the kidney. However, if pyelonephritis occurs in an adult, when active growth of the kidneys is no longer taking place, scarring is rare, although it may occur (Hodson, 1967), and the most valuable radiological finding is inequality in the size of the two kidneys. Little *et al.* (1965) performed intravenous pyelograms in the acute stage of pyelonephritis and found no difference in the size of the kidneys, but on repeating the investigation six months later found shrinkage of the kidney affected by pyelonephritis.

Illustrative Case

W. P. sustained a fracture-dislocation of his first lumbar vertebra on the second, after an accident in 1945. This resulted in a complete paralysis below the 7th thoracic dermatome. Over the ensuing years he had repeated episodes of urinary infection giving rise to shivering and sweating attacks. In 1967 straight X-rays of his abdomen suggested that he had some stones in his right kidney. The conventional intravenous pyelogram of 40 ml of 60 per cent contrast medium on 28 June 1967 (Fig. 4.2 I) showed bilateral hydronephrosis. An infusion pyelogram (Fig. 4.2 II) was performed and showed, in addition, that there was little functioning tissue in the left kidney, presumably due to atrophic pyelonephritis. The nephrogram revealed an almost normal thickness of kidney tissue on the right side. Both ureters filled and were seen to be dilated, suggesting that he had reflux. This was confirmed by a cystogram (Fig. 4.2 III).

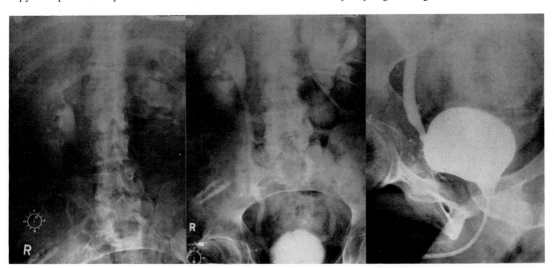

Fig. 4.2. Intravenous pyelography in paraplegia. W.P. sustained a complete traumatic paraplegia below T.7 in 1945. Since injury he had repeated attacks of urinary infection with shivering and sweating.

I. Conventional intravenous pyelogram in June 1967 reveals bilateral hydronephrosis.

II. Subsequent infusion intravenous pyelogram confirms the hydronephroses and in addition shows only a thin rim of functioning renal tissue on the left side, in comparison with the almost normal kidney thickness on the right. The ureters are now well outlined and appear dilated suggesting reflux.

III. Ureteric reflux confirmed by a cystogram.

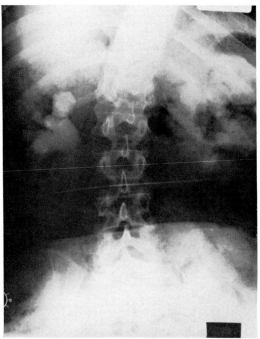

a. S.G. Intravenous pyelogram on admission. Bilateral hydronephrosis. Residual urine 15 oz.

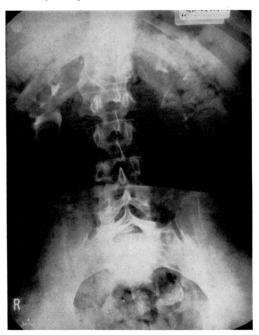

b. S.G. Normal intravenous pyelogram after four months bladder drainage by an indwelling catheter.

FIG. 4.3. Bladder neck obstruction

CYSTOURETHROGRAPHY

The cystourethrogram is an essential part of the radiological investigation of the urinary tract. Ideally, excretionary (descending) cystourethrography, using an image intensifier to reduce the total dose of radiation, and cine radiography should be used. Unfortunately, such facilities are not commonly available. Nevertheless, much valuable information has been obtained by retrograde (ascending) cystourethrography. At the Liverpool Regional Paraplegic Centre the technique described by Damanski and Kerr (1957), and reviewed by Damanski (1965), is used with certain modifications.

Technique

Preliminary films of the bladder area are taken, the bladder is then drained of all urine so that when 4 oz of 10 per cent sodium iodide solution is introduced into the bladder it is not diluted: the catheter is then withdrawn. Antero-posterior and 45° oblique films are taken. The patient is asked to start micturition by whatever means he can, either by abdominal compression, or by triggering off a reflex evacuation by tapping the abdomen. In the last two years, with sufficient patience, most patients have provided an excretionary urethrogram by this technique. Oblique films of the urethra are then taken during the retrograde injection of the contrast medium. Finally, films are taken with the patient straining to see if ureteric reflux is present.

Cystourethrography is of particular value in demonstrating two aspects of bladder dysfunction, obstruction of the outflow of urine at the bladder neck or external sphincter, and the presence of ureteric reflux. It will also demonstrate diverticulae, trabeculation, prostatic diverticula, and vesical stones.

Bladder Neck Obstruction

Obstruction of the bladder outlet plays a significant part in the deterioration of the upper urinary tract (Talbot and Bunts, 1949; Bunts, 1957; Ross *et al.*, 1960; Ross, 1963; Gibbon *et al.*, 1965), and relief of the obstruction improves renal function.

Illustrative Case

S. G. had multiple sclerosis for four years. On admission, although his urine was sterile, there was 15 oz residual urine and the intravenous pyelogram showed gross hydronephrosis with poor secretion. Insertion of a catheter rapidly improved his renal function as shown by the disappearance of the hydronephrosis (Fig. 4.3a and b).

Obstruction occurs at one of two sites, the internal or the external sphincter.

Internal Sphincter. In a patient with paralysis and infection of the bladder, its muscle becomes hypertrophied and the lower lip constitutes a rigid bar or commissure which becomes fibrotic and oedematous. This thick, inelastic tissue is not taken up when the rest of the bladder contracts and constitutes an obstruction to the free passage of urine (Emmett, 1940; Gibbon *et al.*, 1965).

External Sphincter. This is a short area 2–3 cm distal to the prostatic urethra where stricture formation can occur. It is a true stricture and persists despite pudendal neurectomy, and other procedures such as an alcohol block which denervate the pelvic diaphragm. Operations to relieve obstruction at these two sites have resulted in a considerable improvement in the upper renal tract (Emmett, 1940; Ross *et al.*, 1957; Ross *et al.*, 1963; Gibbon *et al.*, 1965). An ascending and descending cystourethrogram gives a good indication of obstruction at the external sphincter, and provides a reliable guide to operation (Fig. 4.4a and b).

It is difficult to assess the relative importance of obstruction at the internal urethral orifice. The ascending cystourethrogram does not give the same information as the excretionary cystourethrogram, as the orifice is normally closed until pulled open by the detrusor action of the bladder, or when the pressure in the bladder is raised by abdominal straining. The findings at retrograde cystourethrography depend on whether the bladder is full or empty, and whether detrusor action is taking place (Fig. 4.4a and b). It is essential to know the state of infection, the catheter status, and the duration of the paraplegia before commenting on the significance of a cystourethrogram (Pritzl and Bors, 1966). This has been confirmed by Ascoli (1967) who always uses the more physiological excretionary cystourethrogram. Gibbon *et al.* (1965) found that there was no reliable pre-operative test to indicate whether a bladder neck resection would be helpful. The presence of a persistent deformity in the form of a ledge or annular stricture was helpful, but it was necessary to feel the texture of the internal sphincter at operation to determine whether resection was indicated. Ascoli (1967) has shown that when more complete studies were carried out, many of the dysfunctions of the bladder previously attributed to internal sphincter derangement, were due to stricture at the external sphincter.

Ureteric Reflux

The other important finding that is revealed by cystourethrography is the presence of ureteric reflux, and for this purpose cine radiology has only a slight

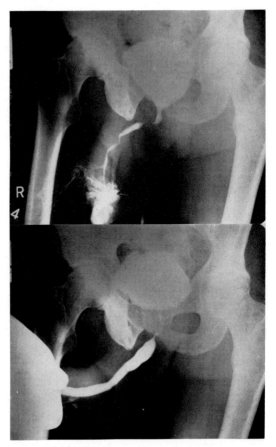

FIG. 4.4. Cystourethrography in paraplegia. T.B. sustained an incomplete traumatic cauda equina lesion in 1957.

Top. Excretory cystourethrogram.
Bottom. Retrograde cystourethrogram.

Note that the radiographs give identical information concerning the external urethral sphincter but completely different information with regard to the internal urethral orifice. On the excretory film the bladder neck is wide open, but appears completely closed on the retrograde film.

advantage over the conventional ascending cystogram. Smith (1966) compared both methods in 145 children. Reflux was detected in 45, and was demonstrated in 25 by both techniques, in 11 by cine radiography alone, and, surprisingly, 9 showed reflux only on the ascending cystogram. He concluded that the cine method yielded slightly better results, but was impressed with the relative efficiency of the standard cystographic method.

Several features contribute to the development of reflux in the paraplegic patient. The paralysis of the 'orthosympathetic innervation of the trigone muscle' in high lesions may play a part, since Bors (1957) has shown that there is a higher incidence of reflux in the upper motor neurone lesion than in the lower motor neurone lesion. Obstruction and infection, leading to panurethritis of the lower end of the urethra as it enters the bladder, is probably more important (Talbot and Bunts, 1949; Talbot, 1958; Cobb and Talbot, 1966; Talbot *et al.*, 1967). Guttmann (1963) showed that in cystograms carried out within twelve months of admission, 37 patients with sterile urine had no reflux, but 2 of 85 patients with infected urine had reflux. Among all the 343 patients in the series, many of whom have been under observation for more than twelve months, the incidence of reflux was 22 per cent.

The development of ureteric reflux has an adverse effect upon the life expectancy of a paraplegic patient. Talbot *et al.* (1967) studied 60 paraplegic patients with reflux and grouped them into those with permanent, and presumably more severe reflux, and those with transient reflux. The patients with permanent reflux had higher blood ureas, a higher incidence of renal calculosis and a higher mortality from renal failure, than those patients with only transient reflux.

Biochemical Tests of Renal Function

The purpose of the kidney is not to make good urine (Samson Wright, quoted by O'Grady), but to maintain the constancy of the internal environment. This is achieved by a combination of glomerular filtration, tubular secretion and reabsorption. De Wardener (1967) gives an up to date description of all forms of renal function tests, and the following section will describe only those routine tests which have been found most useful in assessing renal function in paraplegic patients.

TESTS OF GLOMERULAR FUNCTION

There are several methods of measuring glomerular filtration rate, based on the clearance of a substance from the blood and its detection in the urine. The two most accurate methods of estimating the glomerular filtration rate are the radioactive Vitamin B.12 Clearance and the inulin clearance (*Brit. Med. J.*, 1967). The radioactive Vitamin B.12 clearance requires the use of radioactive isotopes and their measurement by appropriate equipment; the inulin clearance requires an infusion with frequent blood and urine collections: consequently neither test is suitable for routine clinical use.

The creatinine and urea clearances are the most commonly employed clearance tests, and to assess

their use in the evaluation of renal function in paraplegic patients, Doggart and Silver (1963) and Doggart *et al.* (1966) compared the two methods in acute and chronic paraplegic patients. It should be stressed that this was a research procedure with the authors personally collecting the urine specimens and carrying out the majority of the estimations in a research laboratory. Such standards of collection and estimation cannot be obtained in a routine laboratory, especially if the tests are carried out infrequently. In all, 28 patients were studied, 10 of these patients were acute paraplegics and were examined within seventy-two hours of suffering an injury to their spinal cord. Another 18 patients were chronic paraplegics, and were studied between fourteen months and twenty years after injury to their spinal cord or developing a chronic disease of the nervous system. The acute cases did not suffer from renal tract disease secondary to pyelonephritis and their urine was sterile. The chronic cases showed a variety of renal conditions described elsewhere in this monograph. Eleven had amyloidosis, others calculosis, hydronephrosis, and hypertension. Repeated clearance studies at daily intervals by both techniques were carried out to determine the reproducibility of the results, and to assess the value of the clearance studies in determining the prognosis of the patient.

The creatinine and urea clearances do not represent a true glomerular filtration rate as there is some tubular secretion of creatinine and reabsorption of urea. Consequently, the creatinine clearance is always higher than the inulin clearance. This is not a major source of error unless the patient suffers from heavy proteinuria. In these cases, the creatinine clearance is much higher than the inulin clearance, and it is thought that proteinuria in some way enhances the secretion of creatinine into the urine (Berlyne *et al.*, 1964). Tubular reabsorption of urea occurs, but is not constant at all rates of urine flow, being more marked below 2 ml/min. Thus, the urea clearance is always less than the inulin clearance and is particularly inaccurate at low rates of urine flow. There is also evidence of tubular regulation of urea excretion quite independent of the glomerular filtration rate (Samson Wright, 1965).

In order to minimise these errors, the usual procedure is to increase the rate of urine secretion to above 2 ml/min by giving extra oral fluids. However, after any form of acute trauma, urine secretion cannot be increased to above 2 ml/min by giving fluids because of the avid fluid retention. This was reflected in the gross discrepancies found between successive one-hour urea clearances. For these reasons, the urea clearance was not found a satisfactory test of renal function.

The endogenous creatinine clearance does not have these disadvantages, since the clearance does not vary with the rate of urine flow. A further advantage is that as the serum creatinine remains stable for long periods twenty-four hour collections of urine can be used. Graber and Sevitt (1959) used the creatinine clearance as a measure of glomerular filtration rate in oliguric patients following severe burns, and presented evidence to show that the ratio $\frac{\text{creatinine clearance}}{\text{inulin clearance}}$ is the same in a variety of conditions including surgical shock after trauma. The creatinine clearance, therefore, gives reproducible and useful results in the acute stage following injury. In the chronic stage, where the effects of chronic urinary infection were being studied, the urea and creatinine clearances were comparable, gave a useful indication of the degree of renal damage to the patients, and proved of value in assessing the prognosis. This is in accordance with the findings of other workers in the field (Rogers and Bors, 1950; Morales *et al.*, 1956; MaGee, 1957, 1958). Further comments on the above can be seen in Chapter 7, p. 65, concerning renal function tests in amyloidosis.

Accurate collection of urine samples is essential for all clearance tests, and errors are especially likely in paraplegics who may have residual urines up to 300 ml. Even when a catheter is used, it may be difficult to empty the bladder completely, especially in patients with flaccid lesions. It has been shown that the position of the patient (Cook, 1960) and the presence of ureteric reflux (Rosenheim, 1963) can affect the estimation of residual urine in paraplegics. It is recommended in paraplegic patients that a catheter be passed and the clearance studies be performed over a period greater than twelve hours. If the urine is sterile, and passing a catheter thus contraindicated, three successive 24-hour specimens of urine should be collected and the clearances compared.

There is an inverse relationship between the blood urea and the urea clearance, and it is often assumed that if the blood urea is raised, it indicates impaired glomerular filtration. Many other factors can affect the blood urea apart from renal function. It is increased by large amounts of ingested protein, or by protein released within the body after trauma, such as absorption of haematoma at a fracture site. It is reduced by protein deprivation in the treatment of chronic renal failure. A raised blood urea does not necessarily indicate poor renal function. A normal blood urea by no means implies normal renal function without other supporting evidence. If the blood urea is to be used as a screening test, the Azostix (Ames Products) gives fairly accurate results between 20–60 mg/100 ml.

TESTS OF TUBULAR FUNCTION

One of the earliest parts of the kidney to be damaged in chronic pyelonephritis is the renal tubule (Brod, 1962). For this reason, tubular function is assessed separately from glomerular function. The simplest routine test available for tubular function is the ability to concentrate urine in response to water deprivation. The patient is deprived of fluid and food from the previous evening, six specimens of urine are collected at half-hourly intervals from seven o'clock the next morning: the specific gravity is measured by a urinometer and should exceed 1·024. If sugar or protein is present in the urine, the osmolarity should be estimated. The major disadvantages of this test is that deprivation of fluid in patients with chronic renal disease can cause collapse and frequently exacerbates urinary infection.

URINE DILUTION AND WATER ELIMINATION TEST

The converse test, of water loading, has been freely criticised and is seldom used in general medicine for the detection of renal disease since it depends upon—

1. The ability of the patient to drink a litre of water.
2. Absorption of the water is across the bowel wall.
3. The integrity of the pituitary and the adrenal cortex.

The patient is deprived of fluid overnight and usually has no difficulty in drinking a litre of water provided it is given slowly, as most patients have been young fit adults before their injury. Absorption of water across the bowel wall is assessed by studying the serial dilution of the blood with an osmometer. This test has proved valuable in studying patients immediately after an acute cord transection, and patients with amyloid disease and chronic pyelonephritis.

Illustrative Case

M. W. sustained a complete tetraplegia below C.6 after a sugar bag struck him on the back of his neck. He also had a severe head injury and a fractured sternum. His serious injuries and consequent poor general condition made his nursing difficult. He ran a persistent fever after admission, developed haematuria after a week, and his urine became infected. It was not clear whether his fever was due to the chest condition, his head injury, or to his urinary infection. His chest X-ray remained normal, yet despite courses of antibiotics his temperature failed to subside. Investigations of the renal tract were carried out and an infusion intravenous pyelogram two months after injury showed slight dilatation of the lower ureters, suggestive of early back pressure changes. Eventually, after a prolonged course of Penbritin, his fever subsided, his urine became sterile, and his condition steadily improved. A repeat intravenous pyelogram showed that

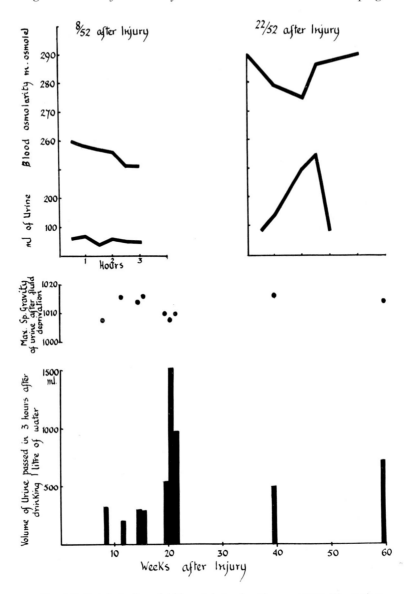

FIG. 4.5. Serial studies of kidney tubular function on M.W. The patient was given one litre of water to drink as the test stimulus. The water is absorbed as reflected by the fall of the serum osmolarity eight weeks after injury, but it is not excreted due to tubular damage. Following improvement in his general health and a prolonged course of Penbritin the water excretion has improved on re-testing twenty-two weeks after injury.

the kidneys were now normal. A series of water absorption tests are illustrated in Fig. 4.5 and show that, although the creatinine clearance remained normal throughout the whole period and he was obviously absorbing water, he could neither concentrate nor excrete it. As time passed, the absorption of the water remained unaltered, but there was a progressive increase in the ability to handle a water load. After twenty-one weeks he was excreting far more than the amount absorbed and had some polyuria. By forty weeks the ability to handle a water load was almost normal, and he was able to concentrate his urine to 1·016.

Summary

Most paraplegic patients die of septic renal complications. The source of this infection is the lower urinary tract from paralysis of the bladder, which leads to impaired emptying of the bladder and consequent obstruction and stasis. Tests should be chosen to demonstrate minor dysfunctions of bladder emptying, as shown by a rise in the residual urine, the development of a persistent infection within the bladder, or dilatation of the lower end of the ureters before irreversible structural changes take place within the kidney.

References

ASCOLI, R. R. (1967) *Int. J. Paraplegia*, **4**, 235.
BAND, D. (1961) *Brit. J. Urol.*, **33**, 361.
BERLYNE, S. M., VARLEY, H., NILWARANGKUR, S. and HOERNI, M. (1964) *Lancet*, **ii**, 874.
BORS, E. (1957) *Urological Survey*, **7**, 177.
BORS, E. (1966) *Med. Serv. J. Can.*, **72**, 666.
BOYCE, W. H., COREY, EL., VEST, S. A. and FRENCH, C. R. (1953) *J. Urol.*, **70**, 605.
BRADLEY, W. E., CHOU, S. N. and FRENCH, L. A. (1963) *J. Neurosurgery*, **20**, 953.
BROD, J. (1962) In, *Renal Disease*, p. 279. Ed. Black, D. A. K. Oxford: Blackwell.
BRITISH MEDICAL JOURNAL (1967) Editorial, p. 455.
BRUMFITT, W. and PERCIVAL, A. (1963) *Proc. 2nd Int. Soc. of Nephrology*, p. 260. Amsterdam: Excerpta Medica Foundation.
BUNTS, C. R. (1957) *Trans. Am. Ass. of G.U. Surgeons*, **49**, 199.
CATTELL, W. R., CURWEN, M. P., SHOOTER, R. A. and WILLIAMS, D. K. (1963) *Brit. med. J.*, **i**, 923.
COBB, O. E. and TALBOT, H. S. (1966) *Int. J. Paraplegia*, **3**, 243.
COMARR, A. E. (1954) *J. Urol.*, **72**, 596.
COMARR, A. E. (1956) *Proceedings of the 5th Annual Clinical Spinal Cord Injury Conference*. Amer. Veterans Adm.
COOK, J. B. (1960) *Proc. roy. soc. Med.*, **53**, 263.
DAMANSKI, M. (1965) *J. Urol.*, **93**, 466.
DAMANSKI, M. (1967) *Hospital Med.*, **2**, 39.
DAMANSKI, M. and GIBBON, N. O. K. (1956) *Brit. J. Urol.*, **28**, 24.
DAMANSKI, M. and KERR, A. S. (1957) *Brit. J. Surg.*, **44**, 398.
DE WARDENER, H. E. (1967) *The Kidney*. 3rd ed. London: Churchill.
DENNY-BROWN, D. and ROBERTSON, E. G. (1933a) *Brain*, **56**, 149.
DENNY-BROWN, D. and ROBERTSON, E. G. (1933b) *Brain*, **56**, 397.
DOGGART, J. R. and SILVER, J. R. (1963) *Int. J. Paraplegia*, **1**, 202.
DOGGART, J. R., GUTTMANN, L. and SILVER, J. R. (1966) *Int. J. Paraplegia*, **3**, 229.
DUBOIS, P. (1876) *Dtsch. Arch. Klin. Med.*, **17**, 148.
EMMET, J. L. (1940) *J. Urol.*, **43**, 692.

FRANKEL, H. and GUTTMANN, L. (1965) *Int. J. Paraplegia*, **3**, 82.
GIBBON, N. O. K. (1950) *Cli. M. Thesis*. Univ. of Liverpool.
GIBBON, N. O. K. (1958) *Brit. J. Urol.*, **30**, 1.
GIBBON, N. O. K. (1966) *3rd Acta Neurol. Scandiv.*, Suppl. 20, **42**, 133.
GIBBON, N. O. K., ROSS, C. J. and DAMANSKI, M. (1965) *Int. J. Paraplegia*, **2**, 264.
GRABER, I. G. and SEVITT, S. (1959) *J. clin. Path.*, **12**, 25.
GUTTMANN, L. (1963) *Int. J. Paraplegia*, **1**, 184.
HARDY, A. G. (1966) *Med. Serv. J. Can.*, **22**, 538.
HEPTINSTALL, R. H. and BRUMFITT, W. (1960) *Brit. J. Exp. Path.*, **41**, 381.
HODSON, C. J. (1959) *Proc. roy. soc. Med.*, **52**, 669.
HODSON, C. J. (1967) *Symposium on Renal Infection*. Lancaster Post Grad. Med. Centre.
HUTCH, J. A. (1966) *J. Urol.*, **96**, 182.
HUTT, M. S. R., CHAMBERS, J. A., MACDONALD, J. R. and DEWARDENER, H. E. (1961) *Lancet*, **i**, 351.
LANCET (1964) Leading Article, **ii**, 77.
LAPIDES, J., SWEET, R. B. and LEWIS, L. W. (1957) *J. Urol.*, **77**, 247.
LEPPER, E. H. (1921) *J. Path. Bact.*, **24**, 192.
LITTLE, P. J., MCPHERSON, D. R. and DEWARDENER, H. E. (1965) *Lancet*, **i**, 1186.
LORD, K. H. and BUNTS, R. C. (1956) *J. Urol.*, **75**, 66.
MCLELLAN, F. C. (1939) *The Neurogenic Bladder*. Springfield, Illinois: Chas. C. Thomas.
MCLEOD, J. W., MASON, J. M. and PILLEY, A. A. (1963) *Lancet*, **i**, 292.
MAGEE, J. H. (1957) *Proceedings of the 6th Annual Clinical Spinal Cord Injury Conference*, p. 32. Amer. Veterans Adm.
MAGEE, J. H. (1958) *Proceedings of the 7th Annual Clinical Spinal Cord Injury Conference*, p. 129. Amer. Veterans Adm.
MILNER, P. F. (1963) *J. clin. Path.*, **16**, 39.
MORALES, P. A. (1967) *The Neurogenic Bladder*. Baltimore: Williams and Wilkins.
MORALES, P. A., SULLIVAN, J. F. and HOTCHKISS, R. S. (1956) *J. Urol.*, **76**, 714.
MUNRO, D. (1936) *New Engl. Med. J.*, **214**, 617.
NESBIT, R. M. (1948) Quoted by Bors, E. (1957).
NYQUIST, R. H. and BORS, E. (1967) *Int. J. Paraplegia*, **5**, 22.
O'GRADY, F. and CATTELL, W. R. (1966) *Brit. J. Urol.*, **37**, 156.
O'GRADY, F. and PENNINGTON, J. H. (1967) *Brit. med. J.*, **i**, 1403.
PRITZL, D. J. and BORS, E. (1966) *J. Urol.*, **96**, 320.
ROGERS, G. W. and BORS, E. (1950) *J. Urol.*, **63**, 100.
ROSE, D. K. (1927) *J. Am. med. Ass.*, **88**, 151.
ROSENHEIM, M. L. (1963) *Brit. med. J.*, **i**, 1433.
ROSS, J. C. (1963) *Symposium on Spinal Injuries*. Edinburgh: Royal College of Surgeons.
ROSS, C. J., DAMANSKI, M. and GIBBON, N. O. K. (1957) *Trans. Amer. Assoc. of G.U. Surgeons*, **49**, 193.
ROSS, C. H., DAMANSKI, M. and GIBBON, N. O. K. (1960) *Brit. J. Surg.*, **206**, 636.
ROSS, C. J., GIBBON, N. O. K. and DAMANSKI, M. (1963) *J. Urol.*, **89**, 692.

SAMSON WRIGHT (1965) *Applied Physiology*. 11th ed. Oxford Med. Public.

SCHIRMER, H. K. A., TAFT, J. L. and SCOTT, W. W. (1966) *J. Urol.*, **96,** 136.

SCHOENBERG, H. W., BEISSWAGER, P., HOWARD, W. J., KLINGENMAIER, H., WALTER, C. F. and MURPHY, J. J. (1964) *J. Urol.*, **92,** 107.

SHELDON, C. H. and BORS, E. (1948) *J. Neurosurg.*, **5,** 385.

SILVER, J. R. and GIBBON, N. O. K. (1968) In press.

SMITH, A. M. (1966) *J. Urol.*, **96,** 49.

SMYTHE, C. A. (1966) *J. Urol.*, **96,** 310.

SOMMER, J. L. and ROBERTS, J. A. (1966) *J. Urol.*, **95,** 502.

SUSSET, J. G., RABINOVITCH, H. and MACKINNON, K. S. (1965) *J. Urol.*, **94,** 113.

TALBOT, H. S. (1958) *J. Amer. med. Ass.*, **168,** 1595.

TALBOT, H. S. and BUNTS, C. (1949) *J. Urol.*, **61,** 870.

TALBOT, H. S., MAHONEY, E. M., JARRETT, E. and COBB, O. E. (1967) *Int. J. Paraplegia*, **5,** 97.

THOMPSON WALKER, J. W. (1917) *Lancet*, **i,** 173.

YEATES, K. (1954) *Brit. J. Urol.*, **26,** 166.

5

Pathology of the Urinary Tract in Chronic Paraplegia: the Effects of Infection and Calculosis

SINCE THE Second World War many papers have been written on different aspects of the urinary tract in paraplegia. They have been confined, almost exclusively, to clinical and therapeutic aspects and only three have been concerned with pathology. Konwaler (1953), in a paper entitled *Renal Pathology in Paraplegia*, divided renal disease into common pyelonephritis, acute pyelonephritis (often suppurative), and necrotising papillitis. He found that renal function tests usually indicated tubular disease, and post-mortem examination showed that the essential renal disease was pyelonephritis. Reingold (1960) gave pathological details of three chronic paraplegics who died from renal failure. They had pure renal amyloidosis, atrophic pyelonephritis without amyloidosis, and obstructive pyelonephritis due to calculi and ascending infection. More recently, Kawaichi and Reingold (1966) described three cases of xanthogranulomatous pyelonephritis in paraplegics: all three had renal calculi. Although pathological details of renal amyloidosis are included in several papers on amyloidosis and paraplegia that are reviewed in the next chapter, none of the authors attempt to describe the place amyloid disease takes in the complex mixture of renal disease found in paraplegics.

No authors appear to have appreciated the wide variety of renal pathology shown in the present study. Much of the difficulty in interpreting the histopathological findings has been in assessing the part played by individual disease processes. As indicated in the previous chapters, pyelonephritis, amyloidosis, calculosis, and hypertension, individually, or in combination, produce bewildering pathological changes. This chapter is concerned with the pathological changes produced by infection and calculosis of the urinary tract, and the changes due to amyloidosis and hypertension will be described in subsequent chapters. Some descriptive overlap is inevitable, however, in clarifying the pleomorphism of the renal disease.

Macroscopic and Microscopic Changes in the Upper Urinary Tract

Most of the descriptions are of the upper urinary tracts of the 86 patients who died from renal failure. However, the kidneys of those patients who died from other causes, and the kidneys removed from patients during life, have also been studied to assess the chronological pattern of renal disease.

The changes in the kidneys will be described in the order in which they are normally studied at necropsy, i.e. external naked-eye appearances, internal naked-eye appearances—on slicing, and histological findings.

I. Macroscopic Changes in the Kidneys—External Appearances

Evidence of old perirenal infection was frequently found, as shown by marked fibrosis and adherence of the perirenal tissues to the kidneys. In three cases, active perinephric abscesses were found at necropsy and there were also three cases of large perinephric haematomata. The perirenal fibrosis was most dense in those patients who had kidney operations during life. Fifty-six separate kidney operations had been performed on the 174 chronic paraplegics in this series, and these are listed in Table 5.1.

TABLE 5.1

Kidney operations in chronic paraplegia

Type of kidney operation	Death related to paraplegia (117 cases)	Death unrelated to paraplegia (57 cases)	Total (174 cases)
Nephrolithotomy	22	1	23
Nephrolithotomy and nephrostomy	11	0	11
Nephrostomy	11	0	11
Nephrectomy	6	0	6
Partial nephrectomy	3	0	3
Nephro-ureterostomy	2	0	2
Totals	55	1	56

From this Table it is evident that dense fibrotic nephrostomy tracts were common at necropsy.

The kidney capsules in those patients who had renal operations or chronic perinephric inflammation were often so adherent that it was impossible to strip them without tearing the underlying kidney tissue. In most cases the capsules were thickened and stripped with some difficulty. Only in the few patients who died from 'pure renal amyloidosis' did the capsules strip easily.

The size of the kidneys varied considerably, and it was unusual to find kidneys of the same size in any one patient. The largest kidneys were found in the cases of acute pyelonephritis and of pure renal amyloidosis. In both diseases, the kidneys were usually equally enlarged. It was, however, more common to find cases in which one kidney was enlarged from amyloidosis and the other contracted and scarred from pyelonephritis (*see* Fig. 3.1).

Kidney weights were also variable. Many of the weights recorded were considered to be unreliable and often too heavy, due to the inclusion of perinephric tissues or accumulations of pus and calculus material in the pelves. For these reasons, no details of kidney weights are included in this chapter.

On stripping the capsule, the external appearance of the kidneys varied considerably. The kidneys from cases of pure renal amyloidosis often showed only a slight diffuse granularity (*see* Fig. 6.3). In cases of acute pyelonephritis, the kidney surfaces were often smooth and showed numerous focal linear small subcapsular abscesses. Histological material from the kidneys was available in 158 of the 174 cases of chronic paraplegia. Of these, 118 (75%) showed evidence of chronic pyelonephritis and this high incidence of chronic renal suppuration was reflected in the external appearances of the kidneys.

In those patients who did not die from renal failure, focal subcapsular scars in the kidneys indicated regions of underlying pyelonephritis. These scars tended to be U-shaped and were often found to be in relation to underlying dilated calyces as described by Smith (1962). The depth and configuration of the scars could often be related to the activity and degree of destruction of renal tissue. Kidneys with active chronic pyelonephritis associated with only moderate tubular destruction showed diffuse, shallow U-shaped scars in contrast to the deeper, more clear-cut scars of kidneys with chronic atrophic ('healed') pyelonephritis. These findings are in agreement with the radiological findings described by Hodson and Wilson (1965).

In patients who died from renal failure, there was often gross contraction and scarring of the kidneys from atrophic chronic pyelonephritis and nephrosclerosis. The kidneys showed not only widespread scarring and coarse granularity but often raised nodular areas corresponding to areas of underlying hypertrophied surviving cortical tubules (Fig. 5.1). In kidneys scarred to this degree, the changes due to secondary hypertension could not be distinguished, and only in the few cases of malignant hypertension were the external appearances of the kidneys altered by the addition of a diffuse 'flea-bitten' haemorrhagic pattern superimposed on the other changes.

II. Macroscopic Changes in the Kidneys—Internal Appearances

On slicing the kidneys, the prominant features were usually abnormalities of the renal pelves and calyces.

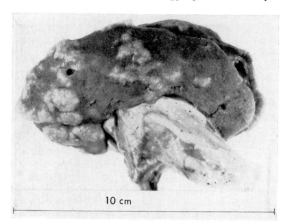

FIG. 5.1. External subcapsular appearance of a kidney from a thirty-six year old paraplegic who died from renal failure due to chronic pyelonephritis, nephrosclerosis, and amyloidosis. There is widespread ischaemic scarring with nodules of hypertrophied tubules in the upper pole.

There was a high incidence of pyo- and hydronephrosis as shown in Table 5.2—

TABLE 5.2

Incidence of pyonephrosis and hydronephrosis in chronic paraplegia

	Death related to paraplegia (117 cases)	Death unrelated to paraplegia (57 cases)	Totals
Pyonephrosis	45 (38%)	8 (15%)	53
Hydronephrosis	22	3	25
Neither	50	46	96

Renal calculi were present in 19 of the 53 pyonephroses (36%). Here, the pyonephroses were usually acute and, on slicing the enlarged kidneys, a huge volume of thick green pus mixed with friable calculi burst out of the grossly dilated pelvi-calyceal systems, leaving only thin rims of surviving renal tissue (Figs. 5.2 and 5.3). These cases illustrate the rapid way in which infection can develop with peripelvic abscesses when there was unrelieved obstruction to the free drainage of urine from the kidneys. It will be shown later that, in patients with kidneys already involved by amyloidosis, temporary urinary obstruction with resulting acute pyelonephritis and pyonephrosis was a frequent terminal complication.

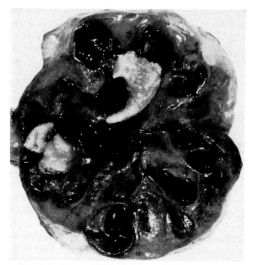

FIG. 5.2. Opened kidney from a forty-seven year old paraplegic who died from lobar pneumonia and renal failure due to calculous pyonephrosis with acute and chronic pyelonephritis in his one surviving kidney. The dilated pelvi-calyceal system has been cleared of pus to reveal several staghorn calculi, one of which was extending down the upper end of the ureter.

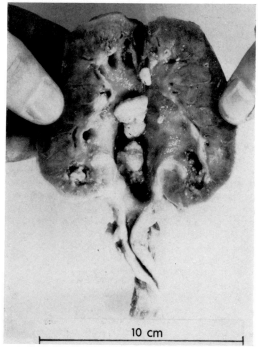

FIG. 5.3. The right kidney of a sixty-two year old paraplegic patient opened to show multiple calculi lying in a thickened pelvi-calyceal system. Death was due to associated amyloidosis and chronic pyelonephritis.

In the cases not associated with calculi, the pyo-nephroses were more often chronic in type and, although the linings of the dilated pelvi-calyceal systems were thickened and shaggy, there was usually a reasonable thickness of surviving renal tissue. There were also a few cases of acute pyonephrosis associated with multiple acute pyelo-nephritic micro-abscesses in the renal tissue. This was a fairly frequent terminal event in cases of severe renal amyloidosis.

In contrast, renal calculi were only present in 5 of the 25 cases of hydronephrosis and gross obstructive hydronephrosis was never seen. The type of hydro-nephrosis most frequently found consisted of only mild dilatation of the pelvi-calyceal system and was probably related to vesico-ureteric reflux, a common finding in paraplegia (Bunts, 1958). Unfortunately, no correlation between reflux in life and the post-mortem findings has been possible in this series.

The kidneys from the few patients who died from acute pyelonephritis showed a swollen renal sub-stance with numerous linear cortical and medullary small abscesses radiating from the hilum. In two post-mortem cases, and in one 'surgical' kidney, there were large acute cortical abscesses suggestive of a haematogenous route of infection.

NECROTISING PAPILLITIS (PAPILLARY NECROSIS)

Konwaller (1953) listed necrotising papillitis in his classification of renal pathology in paraplegia, but this condition was not seen in the 150 post-mortem cases previously reviewed by the author (Tribe, 1963). However, in the further 70 cases analysed for this present study there were 4 cases of bilateral and 2 cases of unilateral necrotising papillitis. Of these, 3 were associated with septicaemia and acute ulcerative endocarditis, and 4 were associated with acute calculous pyonephrosis. Details of the 6 cases are listed in Table 5.3.

Conditions predisposing to necrotising papillitis include pyelonephritis and urinary obstruction, diabetes mellitus, and analgesic abuse (Heptinstall, 1966). Only one of the 6 patients in this series gave a

TABLE 5.3
Papillary necrosis in chronic paraplegia

No	Age	Sex	Level of para-plegia	C* or IC	Survival time (years)	Hydro/ Pyo-nephrosis (H–P)	Renal calculi	Amyloi-dosis	Hyper-tension	Major cause of death
154	53	M	L.2	C	$9\frac{1}{4}$	H	—	—	—	Acute ulcerative endocarditis of aortic valve with widespread chronic PN† and unilateral papillary necrosis
198	46	M	T.10	C	$19\frac{1}{2}$	—	—	+	+	Staphylococcal septicaemia and ulcer-ative endocarditis of mitral valve‡ with renal failure from amyloidosis, acute tubular necrosis, acute PN, and bilateral papillary necrosis
199	47	M	T.12	C	$2\frac{1}{2}$	P	+	—	—	Renal failure from calculous pyo-nephroses with acute and chronic PN, and bilateral papillary necrosis
203	68	M	C.7	IC	$8\frac{1}{2}$	P	+	+	—	Renal failure from calculous pyo-nephrosis, amyloidosis, acute and chronic PN, and unilateral papillary necrosis
216	44	M	C/E	IC	$14\frac{1}{4}$	P	+	+	—	Acute ulcerative endocarditis of the mitral valve with renal failure from amyloidodis, calculous pyoneph-rosis, chronic PN, and terminal papillary necrosis in one surviving kidney
217	32	M	T.7	IC	6	P	+	—	—	Renal failure from acute and chronic PN with bilateral calculosis and papillary necrosis

* C = complete, IC = incomplete.   † PN = pyelonephritis.   ‡ *See* Fig. 2.1.

history of excess intake of Phenacetin, and none of the patients had diabetes. However, the majority of the 174 cases of chronic paraplegia had pyelonephritis, and all had neurogenic urinary obstruction. It is curious, therefore, that no cases of necrotising papillitis were noted prior to 1963, and the explanation may be failure by the pathologists to note this condition at necropsy before the distinctive pathological features of this condition were well known.

Acute terminal pyelonephritis, often with renal calculi or with septicaemia and ulcerative endocarditis, is the probable cause of papillary necrosis in paraplegia.

Irrespective of the changes described so far, naked-eye examination of the sliced kidneys from the patients who died from renal failure showed two main patterns. In cases of almost pure renal amyloidosis, there was an increase in thickness of renal tissue with mild blurring of the cortico-medullary margins. The cortical tissue had a peculiar blotchy white firm waxy appearance characteristic but not diagnostic of amyloid material. In those patients who died from renal failure due to chronic pyelonephritis, the renal tissue was grossly reduced and scarred with an irregular loss of the cortical tissue, usually most marked in relation to the calyces. In these kidneys there was an almost complete loss of differentiation of the cortico-medullary margins. There was an intermediate group with moderate scarring and some irregular loss of renal tissue in

which both chronic pyelonephritis and amyloidosis were found. These appearances are illustrated in Figs. 3.1, 5.4, 5.5, 6.6 and 6.7.

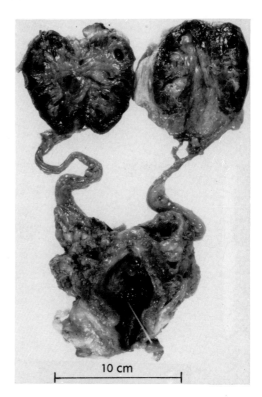

Fig. 5.5. Urinary tract of a thirty-five year old paraplegic patient who died from renal failure, as a result of gross bilateral chronic pyelonephritis with associated severe hypertension. Both kidneys are markedly reduced in size due to pyelonephritic scarring with a moderate terminal pyonephrosis on the left side, and a mild hydronephrosis on the right. The bladder is grossly thickened and contracted and is typical of the changes found in chronic paraplegia.

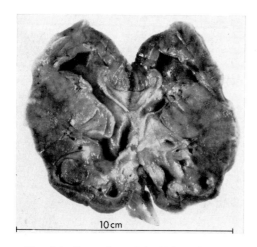

Fig. 5.4. Cut surface of the kidney depicted in Figure 5.1. Note the reduction in size due to pyelonephritis and ischaemic scarring at both poles in relation to the calyces. There is preservation of normal renal thickness in the midzone where the renal tissue has a blotchy white glistening appearance suggestive of amyloidoisis.

III. Microscopic Changes in the Kidneys

Pyelonephritis was the most important of the diseases causing renal failure in this series. Table 3.2 showed that pyelonephritis contributed to renal failure in 71 of 75 patients (95%) in whom kidney material was available for histological study. Apart from causing renal failure *per se*, pyelonephritis also played an important part in producing secondary hypertension, and in the development of renal amyloidosis. The changes in the kidneys due to amyloidosis and hypertension will be dealt with in detail later.

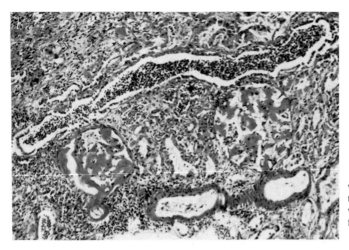

FIG. 5.6. Renal amyloidosis associated with terminal acute pyelonephritis. Note the two glomeruli partially replaced by amyloid with a long dilated tubule lying above them filled with pus cells. Haematoxylin-eosin. ×150.

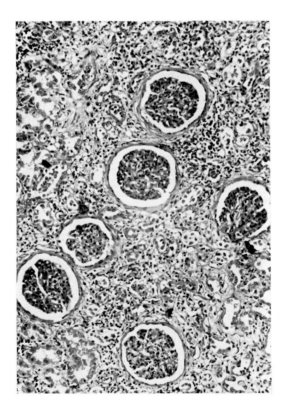

FIG. 5.7. Active chronic pyelonephritis. Note the crowding of the glomeruli with periglomerular fibrosis and preservation of the glomerular tufts. There is a moderate chronic inflammatory cell infiltrate in the interstitial tissues with early destruction and atrophy of the tubules. Haematoxylin-eosin. ×120.

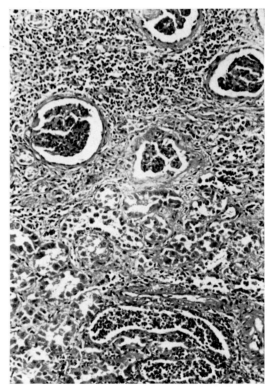

FIG. 5.8. Active chronic pyelonephritis. The features are similar to Fig. 5.7, but there is some sclerosis of the central glomerulus and the tubules at the bottom of the photomicrograph are distended with pus cells. H & E. ×120.

Pyelonephritis

Although the classical papers of Gibson (1928), Staemmler and Dopheide (1930), and Weiss and Parker (1939) established pyelonephritis as a morphological entity, many subsequent writers have failed to agree on the criteria for histological diagnosis. All writers have divided pyelonephritis broadly into acute and chronic stages, and all are agreed as to its focal nature. It is the histological features of chronic pyelonephritis which cause most disagreement. Gall (1961) stated that 'thyroidisation of tubules and concentric periglomerular fibrosis have been considered by many as pathognomonic of pyelonephritis'. Gwynne (1960), however, while recognising that these changes occur, thought that the presence of plasma cells, and or eosinophils, in the interstitial inflammation was diagnostic. Merriam *et al.* (1958) in a study of renal biopsies performed on cases of hypertension undergoing sympathectomy, also considered that plasma cells in the inflammatory infiltrate was the most important single criteria for diagnosing chronic pyelonephritis. Kimmelstiel *et al.* (1961), in a critical review of the morphological aspects of chronic pyelonephritis, concluded that 'an active pleomorphic infiltrate, and particularly accumulation of polymorphs remains the safest criteria for the diagnosis of chronic pyelonephritis'. They thought that all other criteria were relative and required the exclusion of other lesions. Because of this disagreement in histological criteria, the incidence of pyelonephritis in post-mortem series varies considerably. However, the majority of the extensive literature on pyelonephritis is concerned with cases drawn from widely varying age groups usually with different underlying causes and associated diseases. The authors have, therefore, often had the differential diagnosis of pyelonephritis from other renal diseases as an intrinsic and controversial difficulty.

The present series of 220 paraplegics is a highly selected group of patients whose average age at death was around forty, and who all had paralysed bladders with urinary obstruction. It has been frequently shown that obstructive lesions of the urinary tract are the most commonly acquired factors predisposing to renal infection, and the vast majority of these patients had chronic urinary infection during life. Therefore, irrespective of the pathological findings, these patients were obvious candidates for pyelonephritis and, because of their age, they were unlikely to have the congenital or ischaemic renal changes which confuse the histopathologist.

Although the histological features of pyelonephritis in this series did not conform with the specific criteria set down by Kimmelstiel *et al.*, they were basically the same as those described in the early classical papers and the more recent work of Heptinstall (1960, 1966). He divided pyelonephritis into acute, chronic and healed stages, and while agreeing that this is an adequate classification for general use a slightly modified classification has been made to suit the mixed renal pathology seen in this series.

CLASSIFICATION OF PYELONEPHRITIS AS SEEN IN 174 CASES OF CHRONIC PARAPLEGIA

Although there were some intermediate cases, the histological patterns of pyelonephritis in this series could be broadly divided into four groups—

I. Acute pyelonephritis
II. Acute complicating chronic pyelonephritis (this group includes acute pyelonephritis complicating renal amyloidosis)
III. Active chronic pyelonephritis
IV. Atrophic chronic pyelonephritis.

In the following sections no attempt will be made to make a comprehensive description of all the changes produced in these different stages of pyelonephritis. Heptinstall (1966) covers this ground most adequately with a full bibliography. In each group the diagnostic features will be mentioned together with changes, which are either unique to paraplegia or are variations produced by the mixed renal pathology so frequently found in these patients.

I. *Acute Pyelonephritis*

This was characterised by the presence of acute abscesses in the cortex and medulla with destruction of the renal architecture. Only four patients were thought to have died from renal failure due to acute ascending pyelonephritis. This is in marked contrast to the findings in patients who died before the introduction of antibiotics and other modern methods of treatment, when acute renal infection was usually lethal within the first year of paraplegia. One kidney surgically removed from a paraplegic patient contained numerous large cortical abscesses with no evidence of pelvic inflammation. The infection in this case was presumed to be of haematogenous origin and no similar kidneys were found in the post-mortem material.

II. *Acute Complicating Chronic Pyelonephritis*

This group includes cases of renal amyloidosis in which there was histological evidence of terminal acute renal inflammation. Among those who died in renal failure from extensive atrophic chronic pyelonephritis or renal amyloidosis, there were 24 with acute pyelonephritis. In 12, the acute pyelonephritis was associated only with chronic pyelonephritis, usually atrophic in type, and in the other 12 there was associated severe renal amyloidosis. Many of the latter had, in addition, mild or moderate chronic pyelonephritis.

On microscopy, this group was distinguished by the presence of multiple small acute abscesses, containing polymorphs, scattered haphazardly among the chronically diseased renal tissue. Many of the surviving renal tubules were dilated and filled with pus cells (Fig. 5.6). There was often associated acute pyonephrosis and 4 of the 6 cases of papillary necrosis are in this group (*see* p. 38). In the majority of these patients, an ascending acute urinary infection, with or without septicaemia, was the terminal event.

III. *Active Chronic Pyelonephritis*

Characteristically, this was a focal disease and only rarely was it so widespread that it caused renal failure. On microscopy, linear areas of dense interstitial inflammation extending in a V-shaped manner from the medulla to the cortex were found in relation to the macroscopic U-shaped scars. The inflammatory infiltrate was chiefly composed of lymphocytes, but there were usually some plasma cells. Neutrophils were rarely found. There was marked tubular atrophy and interstitial fibrosis in relation to the inflammatory infiltrate. In the cortex, the glomerular tufts were usually intact, but there was always periglomerular fibrosis, and this was a characteristic feature (Figs. 5.7 and 5.8). In the later stages of this condition, some glomeruli became completely hyalinised and, usually at the periphery of the V-shaped inflammatory infiltrate, small

groups of atrophic tubules filled with pink colloid ('thyroid tubules') could be seen (Figs. 5.9 and 5.10). The vessels, even within the most severely involved areas, rarely showed any microscopic changes.

Although the pelvic changes in this group were usually those of a varying sub-epithelial chronic inflammatory cell infiltrate and fibrosis, there were some cases of *xanthogranulomatous pyelonephritis*. This condition, which has only recently been described in any detail (Hooper *et al.*, 1962), consists of a dense inflammatory infiltrate in the tissues around the pelvi-calyceal system with the presence of numerous 'foamy histiocytes' or xanthoma cells, and some cholesterol clefts. On naked-eye examination, there are yellow granulomata surrounding and replacing the pelvi-calyceal linings and extending into the renal tissue. Recently, Kawaichi and Reingold (1966) described 3 cases in paraplegic patients all of whom had staghorn calculi and a predominant *Proteus* urinary infection. Of the 15 cases described by Hooper *et al.*, 12 had renal calculi. This condition was present in this series with or without renal calculi. The most obvious case was in a non-functioning kidney without calculi, removed from a female paraplegic during life (Fig. 6.14). On microscopy, there was a wide band of lipoid-laden macrophages lining the pelvis and calyces, and in many areas these had caused a severe foreign-body reaction with the production of numerous foreign-body multinucleated giant cells. This process is illustrated in Figs. 5.11 and 5.12. In this particular kidney, there was almost confluent, active chronic pyelonephritis throughout the kidney with the formation of many sub-capsular 'local masses' of amyloid. The source of the lipoid material in this

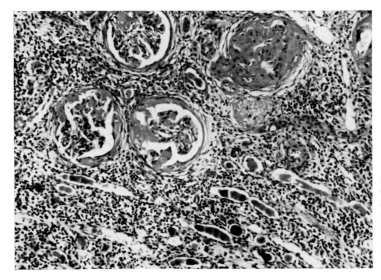

Fig. 5.9. Active chronic pyelonephritis merging into atrophic chronic pyelonephritis. The glomeruli are becoming sclerosed and associated with a dense inflammatory cell infiltrate. The surviving tubules at the bottom of the photomicrograph contain 'thyroid casts'. H & E. ×150.

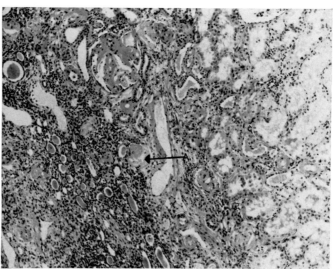

FIG. 5.10. Chronic pyelonephritis and amyloidosis. This photomicrograph illustrates well the focal nature of pyelonephritis. There is a band of atrophic 'thyroid' tubules surrounded by chronic inflammatory cells on the left of the picture sharply demarcated from relatively normal tubules on the right. The glomerulus partially replaced by amyloid at the top of the picture has not been involved in the pyelonephritic process, in contrast to the adjacent small sclerotic glomerulus (*A*) which shows no amyloid deposition. H & E. ×108.

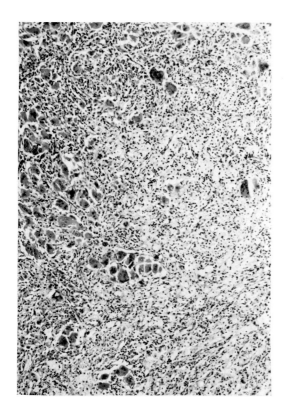

FIG. 5.11. Xanthogranulomatous pyelonephritis. Early stage showing numerous foamy macrophages replacing the renal pelvic lining with early giant cell formation. H & E. ×108.

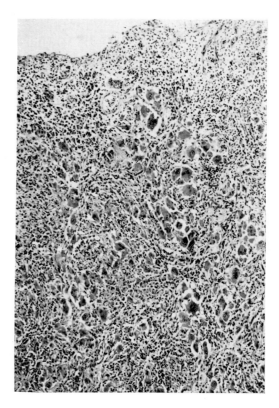

FIG. 5.12. Xanthogranulomatous pyelonephritis. At a later stage than Fig. 5.11. Foamy macrophages now almost absent, with a widespread foreign-body giant cell reaction and early fibrosis. H & E. ×108.

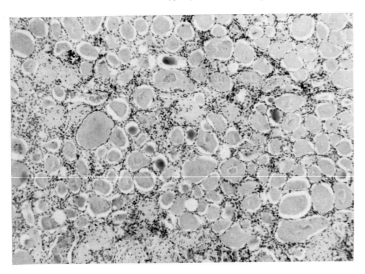

FIG. 5.13. Atrophic chronic pyelone-phritis. Complete 'thyroidisation' of renal tubules. H & E. × 108.

condition is not fully understood, but it is probably of endogenous origin, produced in association with a profuse inflammatory exudate and not directly related to calculus formation.

IV. *Atrophic Chronic Pyelonephritis*

This was the characteristic lesion seen in the kidneys of those patients who died from renal failure solely due to chronic pyelonephritis. In some cases there was a terminal superimposed acute pyelonephritis (Group II). This group can be considered to be the end result of widespread active chronic pyelone-phritis, and cases intermediate between these two groups confirm the progression of active into atrophic chronic pyelonephritis.

The condition occurred in the smallest and most scarred kidneys, and on microscopy there were often large areas in which the glomeruli were either com-pletely hyalinised or had virtually disappeared. The surviving renal tissue was composed of sheets of 'thyroid' atrophic tubules lying around vessels which showed marked intimal thickening (Fig. 5.13). The vascular changes were similar to those described by Weiss and Parker (1939) (Figs. 5.14 and 7.1). There were sometimes small foci of chronic inflammatory cells, but often there was no evidence of active inflammation. Although in many cases this process was widespread throughout the kidney, in others it was still focal in distribution and separated by groups of dilated hypertrophied tubules arranged

FIG. 5.14. Atrophic chronic pye-lonephritis and amyloidosis. The cortical glomeruli are all small and completely sclerosed, and are separated from the medullary 'thyroid' tubules by prominent thickened vessels showing 'en-darteritis fibrosa' and consider-able amyloid infiltration of their muscle coats. No amyloid de-posited either in the sclerotic glomeruli or around the atrophic tubules. H & E. × 108.

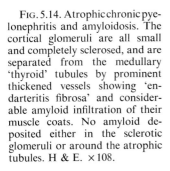
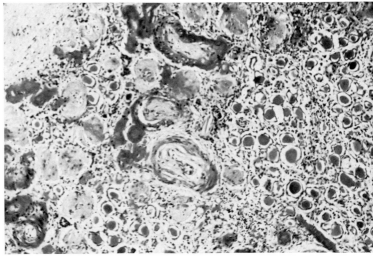

around a few surviving normal glomeruli. In these cases, the appearance of the vessels in the non-involved areas was normal. The comparison between the gross endarteritis fibrosa in the scarred areas with the normal vessels in the adjacent non-scarred areas was striking. However, even when this type of pyelonephritis was associated with hypertension, the vessels in the non-scarred areas showed no appreciable changes unless malignant hypertension had developed. Further comments on renal vascular changes will be made in the chapter on Hypertension in Chronic Paraplegia.

Atrophic chronic pyelonephritis was often associated with amyloidosis. In the cases in which the pyelonephritis was severe, it seemed to have preceded the amyloidosis, since the amyloid was deposited only in those glomeruli which were not hyalinised (Figs. 5.10, 5.14 and 6.12). This picture was in marked contrast to those cases of pure renal amyloidosis in which the glomeruli were all intact, enlarged, and filled with amyloid (Fig. 6.10). Further descriptions of this combination of chronic pyelonephritis and amyloidosis will be made in Chapter 6.

The pelves in this group often showed loss of epithelium and were lined by dense fibrous tissue, lightly infiltrated by chronic inflammatory cells. Occasionally, there were submucosal lymph follicles. In cases when the epithelium was intact, it frequently showed squamous metaplasia and this was usually associated with renal calculosis.

Table 5.4 shows the distribution of these different types of pyelonephritis in the 174 chronic paraplegics

TABLE 5.4
Types of pyelonephritis found in chronic paraplegia

A. 89 PATIENTS DYING FROM RENAL FAILURE

Type of pyelonephritis (PN)	Death related to paraplegia (86 cases)	Death unrelated to paraplegia (3 cases)	Total
No pyelonephritis	4*	2†	6
Group I			
Acute pyelonephritis	4	0	4
Group II			
Acute-chronic pyelonephritis (12) ⎱	24	1‡	25
Acute PN with amyloidosis (12) ⎰			
Group III			
Active chronic PN	5	0	5
Group IV			
Atrophic chronic PN	38	0	38
No histology available	11	0	11

* These four patients died from either pure renal amyloidosis (2 cases), or renal amyloidosis and hypertension (2 cases).
† These patients died from chronic glomerulonephritis.
‡ This patient died from malignant hypertension unrelated to paraplegia, with a terminal unilateral acute pyelonephritis.

B. 85 PATIENTS DYING FROM CAUSES OTHER THAN RENAL FAILURE

Type of pyelonephritis (PN)	Death related to paraplegia (31 cases)	Death unrelated to paraplegia (54 cases)	Total
No pyelonephritis	10	19	29
Group I			
Acute pyelonephritis	1	1	2
Group II			
Acute-chronic pyelonephritis	3	4	7
Group III			
Active-chronic PN	7	15	22
Group IV			
Atrophic chronic PN	8	12	20
No histology available	2	3	5

studied. Although some cases showed kidneys with pyelonephritis at different stages, these have been placed in one group or another according to which stage predominated.

Comparison between the two parts of Table 5.4 shows several points.

I. Acute pyelonephritis, which took such a toll of the First World War paraplegics, now plays only a minimal part in the major causes of death in paraplegics in Spinal Centres. However, it often appears to be the terminal event when the kidneys are severely damaged by chronic pyelonephritis or amyloidosis after acute obstruction of the lower urinary tract.

II. Atrophic chronic pyelonephritis predominates in those cases who died from renal failure, and active chronic pyelonephritis predominates in those cases who did not die from renal failure.

III. Although this table only indicates the histological type of pyelonephritis and not its extent, it confirms the histological impression that active chronic pyelonephritis progresses to atrophic chronic pyelonephritis. This progression depends upon treatment, drainage, calculi, and long-term antibiotics, but it must be emphasised that there is no such condition as 'healed' pyelonephritis, in the sense that the renal tissue returns to normal as the lung does after classical pneumococcal lobar pneumonia. Every attack of pyelonephritis eventually results in the destruction of a portion of irreplaceable renal tissue, and this insidious destruction of functioning nephrons eventually leads to the histological picture recognisable as atrophic chronic pyelonephritis. Although atrophic chronic pyelonephritis appears to be especially lethal, many cases had amyloidosis and others developed hypertension prior to death. In only 17 patients was chronic pyelonephritis considered to be the sole cause of renal failure (*see* Table 3.2).

An attempt was made to assess the severity and extent of chronic pyelonephritis in each case, on the following grades—

± Very occasional sub-cortical scars containing hyalinised glomeruli, usually with some cellular infiltration. These changes were not always diagnostic of pyelonephritis.

+ Small focal areas of either active or atrophic chronic pyelonephritis.

++ The majority of these cases had fairly widespread focal active chronic pyelonephritis. A few cases with widespread, but still focal, atrophic chronic pyelonephritis were also included.

+++ Virtually complete involvement of the kidneys by atrophic chronic pyelonephritis.

Using this method of grading, the amount of chronic pyelonephritis in 174 chronic paraplegics is shown in Table 5.5.

Of the 158 cases with kidney tissue available for microscopy, 124 (78%) showed evidence of pyelonephritis. (As most of the 16 cases with no histological material were patients who died from renal failure

TABLE 5.5
Extent of chronic pyelonephritis in 174 chronic paraplegics

Grade of extent of CPN	Death related to paraplegia (117 cases)	Death unrelated to paraplegia (57 cases)	Total
Nil	13	21	34
± and +	30	18	48
++	26	13	39
+++	35	2	37
No kidney material available for histology	13	3	16

between 1945 and 1950, the true incidence is probably between 80–90 per cent.) As only a few of these patients died before the advent of modern antibiotics, the figures show that this treatment is not a panacea for infections of the urinary tract. Although paraplegic patients live longer now than in the pre-antibiotic era, renal inflammation still plays a very important part in their ultimate death.

Renal Adenomata

An incidental finding in some of the kidneys in this series was the presence of small renal adenomata. With the exception of one large clear cell adenoma (2 cm diameter) found in a 'pure amyloid kidney' these adenomata were all of the papillary type. They varied in size from being just visible to the naked eye, down to as large as two dilated tubules (Figs. 5.15 and 5.16). As the photomicrographs show, they are composed of papillary metaplastic tubular epithelial cells. None of these tumours showed cyst formation and in none was there any attempt at clear cell differentiation.

INCIDENCE

Of the 104 kidneys available for histological study from the 117 patients who died from causes related to their paraplegia, 22 (21%) showed one or more renal adenomata. In contrast, only 2 of the 54 kidneys available for study from the 57 patients who died from causes unrelated to their paraplegia showed adenomata. The majority of the adenomata were found in the kidneys of those paraplegics who died from renal failure. Although usually only one

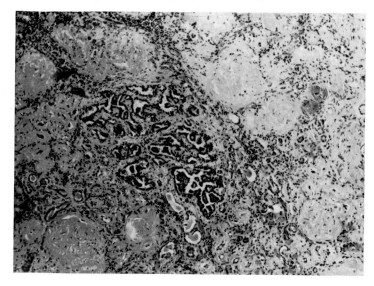

FIG. 5.15. Groups of metaplastic tubules starting to form a papillary renal adenoma in a kidney involved by amyloidosis and atrophic chronic pyelonephritis. H & E. ×120.

or two tumours were found in each case, the kidneys from 2 cases showed multiple adenomata and in five sections from the kidneys of one patient twenty adenomata of varying size were seen. If more histological material had been studied, the true incidence of these tumours might be considerably higher.

AETIOLOGY

Of the 24 cases showing renal papillary adenomata, all showed severe chronic pyelonephritis. Associated amyloidosis was seen in 12 cases, and 10 had proven clinical and pathological hypertension. These tumours appear to occur mainly in kidneys scarred from chronic pyelonephritis. Other authors have

noted this association, but have usually stressed the coexisting arteriosclerotic renal changes. Fuchsman and Angrist (1948) found 79 benign renal tumours in 3,456 consecutive post-mortems, and in 73 per cent the kidneys showed sclerotic changes of some degree. Childs and Waterfall (1953) quoted the former paper, and that of Newcomb (1937) who found 147 adenomata in 84 kidneys. They stated that all authors emphasise the association of adenomas with arteriosclerotic changes in the kidney. Willis (1960) stated that the kidney almost always shows distinct evidence of arteriosclerotic or chronic nephritic changes. He also thought that these tumours arose from the epithelium of hyperplastic convoluted

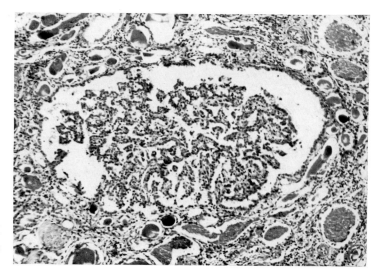

FIG. 5.16. A typical papillary renal adenoma in a kidney involved by severe atrophic pyelonephritis. H & E. ×108.

tubules, and in some cases traced continuity of adenomatous epithelium with renal tubules. All these authors found their adenomata in middle or old age and Willis considered them to be definitely pre-malignant.

The adenomata found in the kidneys in this series differed from those described by other authors in occurring in a younger age group, being usually microscopic, only of the papillary type and showing no tendency to malignant change. No cases of renal carcinoma occurred in this series, and these tumours appear to be the result of benign metaplastic proliferation of hyperplastic tubules occurring in kidneys scarred from extensive chronic pyelonephritis.

CHANGES IN THE URETERS

These were 19 operations during life on the ureters of the 174 chronic paraplegics in this series—

Ureterolithotomy	7
Ureterostomy	6
Ureterolysis	3
Uretero-cystectomy for carcinoma of the ureter	1
Transplantation of the ureters for carcinoma of the bladder	2

At necropsy, ureteric calculi were found in only 4 cases. Macroscopically the ureters usually showed some degree of dilatation associated with thickening and fibrosis of their walls. In some cases of acute pyonephrosis there were associated pyoureters, but this was uncommon.

Talbot (1958) investigated the role of the ureter in the pathogenesis of ascending pyelonephritis and considered that inflammatory changes in the ureteral wall, as well as direct inflammation through the lumen of the ureter, played a large part in producing pyelonephritis after obstruction of the urinary tract. The relationship of the ureters to bladder and kidney infection has previously been discussed (*see* p. 29).

In this series, only a few ureters were available for histological study and these were usually taken from cases of long-standing urinary tract infection. They showed a non-specific fibrous thickening of the ureteric wall with variable amounts of chronic inflammatory cell infiltration in the sub-mucosa. Further studies are needed on the ureters of paraplegics who die from non-renal causes, but who show evidence of early pyelonephritis, to give a better understanding of the pathogenesis of pyelonephritis.

Macroscopic and Microscopic Changes in the Lower Urinary Tract

In contrast to the varied renal pathology found in this series, the pathological changes in the bladders of the chronic paraplegics presented a fairly uniform picture.

Without exception, all 174 chronic paraplegics in this series had chronic urinary tract infection due to a mixture of pathogenic bacteria. In the majority of patients, this infection was persistent from soon after the onset of their paraplegia to the time of death. *Suprapubic cystotomy* was performed as an emergency on 83 of these patients soon after the onset of their paraplegia. These were closed after varying intervals. In 43 patients, the cystotomies were present for more than two years and, in 13, they remained open for more than five years. There was a much higher proportion of long standing cystotomies among the patients who died from causes related to their paraplegia, and, although it is recognised that this form of treatment destroys the normal bladder physiology and potentiates infection, it does allow free urinary drainage without obstruction and back pressure effects on the kidney. It should be remembered that many of the longest surviving patients, who had initially poor treatment by modern standards, had suprapubic cystotomies and this form of treatment should be reconsidered in certain cases.

Bladder calculi also played a part in maintaining urinary infection. A total of 36 bladder operations were performed during life for the removal or crushing of calculi, and in 15 cases calculi were found in the bladder at necropsy.

Macroscopic Findings

The usual naked-eye appearance of the chronic paralysed bladder at necropsy, was of a thick-walled contracted viscus with variable amounts of perivesical fibrosis (Fig. 5.5). Any operations during life, suprapubic cystotomy or lithotomy, greatly increased the perivesical fibrosis and, in some cases, a suprapubic sinus from an unclosed cystotomy led to an even more contracted bladder than usual. In 3 patients there was active perivesical inflammation with the formation of extra-peritoneal pelvic abscesses, and in one the pelvic abscess had ruptured into the peritoneal cavity producing a pelvic peritonitis.

The bladder usually contained cloudy purulent urine, with thickening and granularity of the mucosa.

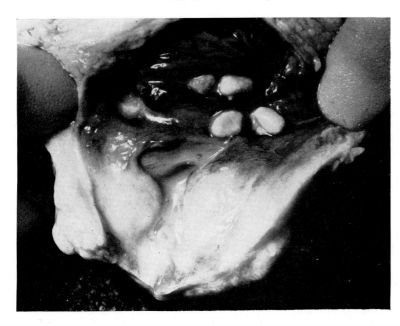

FIG. 5.17. Bladder calculi in chronic paraplegia. Note the multiple, small, oval friable calculi, the severe congestion of the mucosa and the scarring of the prostatic urethra. This patient also had bilateral renal calculi.

If calculi were present, they were usually multiple, oval and friable (Fig. 5.17). Trabeculation of the mucosa, as seen in chronic prostatic obstruction, was rarely found, but some chronically inflamed bladder diverticula were present.

These changes were in marked contrast to the bladders found at necropsy in the 46 cases of acute paraplegia. Although there were some instances of mild cystitis, none of these bladders were thickened and these usually showed no naked-eye differences from bladders seen in non-paraplegic patients. This contrast reflects the good results obtainable by intermittent catheterisation, the standard treatment of the paralysed bladder at Stoke Mandeville Hospital for many years (Guttmann and Frankel, 1966).

Microscopic Findings

Representative histological sections of the bladder were available from the majority of cases. These usually showed loss of the epithelial lining (probably due to post-mortem autolysis), with slight to moderate infiltration of the sub-mucosa by chronic inflammatory cells. Sub-mucosal lymph follicles were occasionally found. The sub-mucosal layer was invariably thickened due to fibrosis, and this extended throughout the muscle coats which were thickened from fibrosis and muscle hypertrophy. Evidence of acute cystitis was only rarely encountered and no chronological pattern of bladder infection was obtained.

In this series, 4 patients died as a direct result of carcinoma of the bladder, and another patient had an extensive carcinoma, confined to the bladder, which contributed to his death from renal amyloidosis (Table 5.6).

Kawaichi (1960) described 4 cases of carcinoma of the bladder in patients below the age of fifty, occurring over fifteen years in 1,600 paraplegics at the Veterans Administration Hospital, Long Beach, California. These patients had all survived more than fourteen years after the onset of paraplegia, and they all had chronic urinary infection.

Melzak (1966) reported 11 cases of bladder cancer observed at the National Spinal Injuries Centre, Stoke Mandeville Hospital, among 3,800 paraplegic and tetraplegic patients treated since 1944. These included the post-mortem cases listed in Table 5.6. The diagnosis was made from thirteen to forty-two years after the onset of paraplegia, and the only common aetiological factor in all these patients was long-standing bladder infection. Early diagnosis of carcinoma of the bladder in paraplegics is now being attempted with some success by routine cytological examinations of the urine (Wolfendale, 1968).

It seems fairly certain that persistent chronic infection of the paralysed bladder can lead to carcinoma, often in relatively young patients. The majority of these tumours are either squamous or show squamous metaplasia (Fig. 5.18). It is surprising that, apart from one case with a transitional carcinoma of the lower end of the ureter, no other

TABLE 5.6
Carcinoma of the bladder in chronic paraplegia

No.	Age	Sex	Spinal lesion*	Time since onset of paraplegia	Type and extent of carcinoma of the bladder	Part played by carcinoma in cause of death
79A	33	M	T.12.C	13¼ years	Localized transitional cell carcinoma with some squamous metaplasia. Spread to local lymph nodes and caused terminal peritonitis.	Major
117	38	F	T.5.C	14½ years	Extensive poorly differentiated transitional cell carcinoma with areas of squamous metaplasia. Spread locally and into abdominal cavity.	Major
155	36	M	T.4.C	19 years	Extensive well differentiated squamous carcinoma. Spread locally into the pelvis with scanty haematogenous metastases.	Major
218	54	M	C.8.IC	20 years	Extensive anaplastic squamous carcinoma. Widespread lymphatic spread in the abdomen and thorax.	Major
193	53	M	T.11.C	18 years	Diffuse poorly differentiated transitional cell carcinoma confined to the bladder.	Contributory

* C = complete spinal paralysis and IC = incomplete spinal paralysis.

carcinomata of the upper urinary tract have been found in this series or in the literature.

The remainder of the lower urinary tract was not studied in detail in this series. The prostate usually showed no gross abnormalities. On microscopy there was often some degree of chronic prostatitis, and in some cases the tubules were filled and dilated with pus cells and there was early abscess formation.

Penoscrotal diverticula and fistulae are frequent complications of male paraplegics. Comarr and Bors (1951), discussing the pathological changes in the urethra of paraplegic patients, found an incidence of 6·9 per cent penoscrotal fistulae in 619 paraplegics. No post-mortem material from the penile urethra was available from this series, but surgical specimens of excised fistulous tracts showed changes similar to those described by these authors.

Urinary Tract Calculosis

The paraplegic patient is specially liable to develop calculosis of the urinary tract for several reasons—

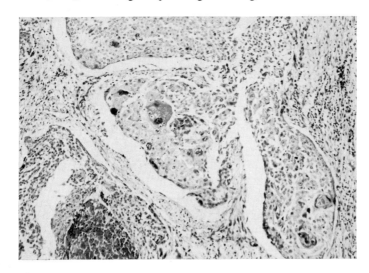

FIG. 5.18. Section from a carcinoma in the bladder of a chronic female paraplegic patient, Case no. 117 (details in Table 5.6). The tumour is basically a transitional cell carcinoma with areas of squamous metaplasia and attempted keratin formation. H & E. ×108.

1. Immobilisation leads to osteoporosis, hypercalcinosis and urinary stasis.
2. Paralysis of the bladder leads to impaired free drainage of urine with a high incidence of infection.
3. The use of sulphonamides and indwelling catheters may serve as foci for stone formation.
4. Pyonephrosis in patients with high spinal cord lesions may be a 'silent' condition, and this leads to delay in the diagnosis of the frequently associated calculi.

The apparent inconsistency in these tables is explained by the frequent operative removal of urinary tract calculi during life. Calculi were usually removed when detected in the bladder or ureters, but a more conservative approach was employed with regard to renal calculi. Table 5.8 shows the number of operations performed on the urinary tracts of the 174 chronic paraplegics in this series, and is subdivided to show the proportion of operations performed for the removal of calculi.

Of the 111 operations performed on the urinary

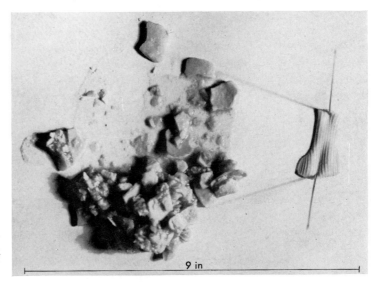

FIG. 5.19. Part of the balloon of a Foley catheter (coated with egg shell calculi) removed from the bladder of a paraplegic patient.

Although these factors produce a higher incidence of urinary tract calculosis in paraplegics, the pathological findings are similar to those found in non-paraplegics, apart from a tendency for calculi in the paralysed bladder to be multiple and of the egg-shell variety. This has been noted by Comarr *et al.* (1962) to be related to the presence of indwelling catheters of the Foley type, and is sometimes associated with a burst balloon. Figure 5.19 illustrates a piece of balloon and egg-shell calculi removed from a tetraplegic.

Analysis of the material in this post-mortem series suggests that renal calculosis must have played a part in the high incidence of renal failure. Without a comparison with the incidence of calculi in the surviving paraplegics at this Centre, it has not been easy to assess the importance of calculosis in renal disease in paraplegia. Analysis of the number of patients in this series in whom calculi were found, both during life and at necropsy (Table 5.7), gives some idea of the extent of urinary tract calculosis, and provides some information as to its importance.

tracts of the 174 chronic paraplegics in this series, 73 per cent were for removal of calculi and, in several patients, repeated lithotomies had to be performed. When the high incidence of renal failure in the 117 patients who died from causes related to their paraplegia is recalled, it suggests that calculosis of the urinary tract must have played a significant part in the aetiology of renal failure. It also shows that, once operative procedures for any reason are required on the urinary tract of a paraplegic, the ultimate prognosis is poor.

Comarr *et al.* (1962) reviewed renal calculosis in 1,507 patients with traumatic cord lesions from the Spinal Cord Injury Service of the Veterans Administration Hospital, Long Beach, California between 1946 and 1960, and found 124 (8·2%) had unilateral or bilateral renal calculosis. Of these, 18 had died; 15 in uraemia including 3 cases of amyloidosis. Damanski (1963) in an article on *Stone Disease in Paraplegia* ended his conclusions with a warning: 'when a stone has developed in the kidney in paraplegia, the long-term prognosis is not good'.

TABLE 5.7
Urinary tract calculosis in 174 fatal cases of chronic paraplegia

A. PATIENTS WITH CALCULI DETECTED DURING LIFE*

Site of calculi	Death related to paraplegia (117 cases)	Death unrelated to paraplegia (57 cases)	Total
Kidney	41	3	44
Ureter	12	4	16
Bladder	22	5	27

B. PATIENTS WITH CALCULI FOUND AT POST-MORTEM

Site of calculi	Death related to paraplegia (117 cases)	Death unrelated to paraplegia (57 cases)	Total
Kidney	32	7	39
Ureter	0	4	4
Bladder	8	7	15

* Some patients had multiple calculi in one site at different times during their life, but these were only counted once in compiling this Table.

Although there is evidence from different Spinal Centres that the incidence of calculosis in paraplegia is falling sharply with modern methods of treatment (Guttmann, 1953; Comarr, 1955; Comarr *et al.*, 1962; Damanski, 1963), there is little doubt from the findings in this series, and those of other authors, that renal calculosis is a dangerous and potentially lethal condition in paraplegia.

TABLE 5.8
Operations performed on the urinary tracts in 174 chronic paraplegics

Site of operation	Death related to paraplegia (117 cases)	Death unrelated to paraplegia (57 cases)	Total	No. and percentage of operations for removal of calculi
Kidney	55	1	56	34 (61%)
Ureter	18	1	19	13 (68%)
Bladder	34	2	36	34 (95%)
Total	107	4	111	81 (73%)

References

BUNTS, R. C. (1958) *J. Urol.*, **79**, 747.
CHILDS, P. and WATERFALL, W. B. (1953) *Brit. J. Urol.*, **25**, 187.
COMARR, A. E. (1955) *J. Urol*, **74**, 447.
COMARR, A. E. and BORS, E. (1951) *J. Urol.*, **66**, 355.
COMARR, A. E., KAWAICHI, G. K. and BORS, E. (1962) *J. Urol.*, **87**, 647.
DAMANSKI, M. (1963) *Int. J. Paraplegia*, **1**, 149.
FUCHSMAN, J. J. and ANGRIST, A. (1948) *J. Urol.*, **59**, 167.
GALL, E. A. (1961) *Bull. N.Y. Acad. Med.*, **37**, 367.

GIBSON, A. G. (1928) *Lancet*, **ii**, 903.
GUTTMANN, L. (1953) *Medical History of the Second World War. Surgery*, pp. 422–515. London: H.M.S.O.
GUTTMANN, Sir L. and FRANKEL, H. (1966) *Int. J. Paraplegia*, **4**, 63.
GWYNNE, J. F. (1960) *Aust. Ann. of Med.*, **9**, 150.
HEPTINSTALL, R. H. (1960) *Recent Advances in Pathology*. 7th ed., Chapter 4. London: J. & A. Churchill.
HEPTINSTALL, R. H. (1966) *Pathology of the Kidney*. Boston: Little, Brown.
HODSON, C. J. and WILSON, S. (1965) *Brit. med. J.*, **ii**, 191.

HOOPER, R. G., KEMPSON, R. L. and SCHLEGEL, J. U. (1962) *J. Urol.*, **88**, 585.

KAWAICHI, G. K. (1960) *Proceedings of the 9th Annual Clinical Spinal Cord Injury Conference*, p. 104. Amer. Veterans Adm.

KAWAICHI, G. K. and REINGOLD, I. M. (1966) *Canad. Serv. med. J.*, **22**, 559.

KIMMELSTIEL, P., KIM, O. J., BERES, J. A. and WELL-MAN, K. (1961) *Amer. J. Med.*, **30**, 589.

KONWALER, B. E. (1953) *Proceedings of the 2nd Annual Clinical Spinal Cord Injury Conference*, p. 42. Amer. Veterans Adm.

MELZAK, J. (1966) *Int. J. Paraplegia*, **4**, 85.

MERRIAM, J. C., SOMERS, S. C. and SMITHWICK, R. H. (1958) *Circulation*, **17**, 243.

NEWCOMB, W. D. (1937) *Proc. roy. Soc. Med.*, **30**, 113.

REINGOLD, I. M. (1960) *Proceedings of the 9th Annual Clinical Spinal Cord Injury Conference*, p. 112. Amer. Veterans Adm.

SMITH, J. F. (1962) *J. clin. Path.*, **15**, 522.

STAEMMLER, M. and DOPHEIDE, W. (1930) *Virchows Arch. path. Anat.*, **277**, 713.

TALBOT, H. S. (1958) *J. Amer. Med. Ass.*, **168**, 1595.

TRIBE, C. R. (1963) *Post-mortem Findings in Paraplegic Patients*. D.M. Thesis. Oxford.

WEISS, S. and PARKER, F. (1939) *Medicine (Baltimore)*, **18**, 221.

WILLIS, R. A. (1960) *Pathology of Tumours*. London: Butterworths.

WOLFENDALE, MARGARET R. (1968) Personal communication.

6

Amyloidosis in Chronic Paraplegia

THERE IS virtually no mention of the association of amyloidosis with paraplegia in current textbooks; yet chronic sepsis, in the form of pressure sores, osteomyelitis, and urinary tract infection, is the most serious complication of chronic paraplegia. Therefore, it is not surprising that secondary amyloidosis played such a large part in the cause of renal failure in this series.

The first reference which mentioned the association of amyloidosis with paraplegia was that of Hilton Fagge in 1876. He described 244 cases of lardaceous disease seen between 1855–75, most of which were due to syphilis or chronic suppuration. Among the latter, he attributed 2 cases to bedsores after fractures of the spine. One year later, Howship Dickinson (1877) described 66 cases, one of which was due to 'long and continued bedsores'.

Apart from these early papers, no references described amyloidosis due to bedsores, with or without paraplegia, until 1949. There are occasional references to amyloidosis in association with chronic renal suppuration, a condition that often complicates paraplegia. Bell (1933) described 65 cases of amyloidosis and attributed 2 to pyonephrosis. He also included 2 cases due to secondary infection following transverse myelitis, but gave no further details. Rosenblatt (1933) described 125 cases of amyloidosis, of which only 15 were of non-tuberculous origin. He thought 4 of the latter cases were due to pyonephrosis.

This dearth of references is because paraplegics, before the Second World War, died before they could develop amyloidosis. Now that paraplegics live for many years, amyloidosis occurs after long periods of chronic suppuration of bone (due to decubitus ulceration) and of the urinary tract. When Thompson and Rice described 4 cases in 1949, they claimed the only previous reference to amyloidosis and spinal cord injury was that of Fagge in 1876. Since this paper, several other authors have described small numbers of cases and these are tabulated in Table 6.1.

COMMENTS ON MODERN REFERENCES TO AMYLOIDOSIS AND PARAPLEGIA (TABLE 6.1)

I. These references can be divided into two main groups—

A. Authors describing a few cases in detail without attempting to estimate the incidence of amyloidosis in paraplegia (Nos 1, 2, 3, 5, 7, 12, 13 and 14).

B. Authors who included the incidence of amyloidosis in paraplegia in mortality statistics with only brief pathological comments (Nos 4, 6, 8, 9, 10 and 15).

The article of Briggs (1961) is unique. He included 24 cases of amyloidosis due to septic complications of paraplegia in a general study of amyloidosis. However, this paper was chiefly concerned with primary amyloidosis and there are only scanty details of the paraplegic cases.

The article of Doggart et al. (1966) is also of special interest. In a study of renal function tests in paraplegics and quadriplegics the diagnosis of amyloidosis was established by means of rectal biopsy. Dr J. R. Silver, who was a co-author in this paper, has amplified this material with more recent experience both in this chapter and in Chapter 4.

Only the author, who in the present series includes the 48 cases first described in 1963 with 17 additional cases, has combined detailed descriptions of the pathological changes found at post-mortem with analysis of the incidence and systemic effects of amyloidosis.

II. All authors who have discussed the aetiology of amyloidosis have incriminated decubitus ulceration, usually with associated osteomyelitis, as the chief causal factor. Although urinary tract suppuration is frequently thought to be a contributory cause, no authors claimed this to be the only cause of amyloidosis.

III. These papers give a clear indication of the rapidity with which amyloidosis may develop in

TABLE 6.1

Modern references to amyloidosis and paraplegia

	Authors	Cases with amyloidosis	No. of necropsies	Survival rate Shortest	Longest	Aetiology
1.	Thompson and Rice, 1949	4	—	—	—	Decubitus ulcers Urinary tract infection Osteomyelitis
2.	Bowman and Redfield, 1951	4	—	11 months	27 months	Decubitus ulcers Urinary tract infection
3.	Newman and Jacobson, 1953	6	—	—	—	Decubitus ulcers
4.	Reingold, 1953	3	25	4 years	18 years	Pyelonephritis Decubitus ulcers
5.	Moses, 1954	4	—	$2\frac{3}{4}$ years	9 years	Decubitus ulcers
6.	Comarr, 1954 and 1955a	6	73 deaths	11 months	$17\frac{1}{2}$ years	Osteomyelitis (major) Decubitus ulcers
7.	Box, 1957	4	29	14 months	17 years	Decubitus ulcers (major) Chronic pyelonephritis (minor)
8.	Dietrick and Russi, 1958	12	51	24 months	53·8 months (average)	All with decubitus ulcers
9.	Nyquist, 1960	13	149 deaths	3 years	15·3 years (average)	All with chronic osteo-myelitis due to decu-bitus ulcers
10.	Breithaupt *et al.*, 1961	4	40	—	—	—
11.	Briggs, 1961	24	24	—	—	Chronic decubitus ulcers Chronic pyelonephritis Chronic osteomyelitis
12.	Maglio and Potenza, 1963	2	—	11 years	14 years	Decubitus ulcers Osteomyelitis Urinary tract infection
13.	Vasquez, 1963	1	—	8 years		Urinary tract infection
14.	Malament *et al.*, 1965	4 2 alive	2	5 years	19 years	Osteomyelitis due to decubitus ulcers
15.	Dalton *et al.*, 1965*	26	89	11·3 years (average)		Decubitus ulceration
16.	Doggart *et al.*, 1966†	11	3	—	—	—
17.	Nyquist and Bors, 1967	24	99	—	—	Decubitus ulcers
18.	Tribe, 1963a and 1963b	48	122	2 years	$19\frac{1}{2}$ years	Discussed later
19.	Present series	65	174	1·5 years	25 years	Discussed later

* This article included the 12 cases previously reported by Dietrick and Russi in 1958 (No 8).
† This article written on renal function tests in paraplegics and tetraplegics from Stoke Mandeville Hospital, included 11 cases of amyloidosis. The 3 necropsies are included in the present series (No 19).

paraplegic patients. Two authors report cases which developed within eleven months of the onset of paraplegia.

The findings of these authors will be quoted and compared with this series in the remainder of this chapter.

Incidence

POST-MORTEM

Apart from the findings of Dalton *et al.* (1965), Nyquist and Bors (1967), and those of the present series, no authors have described the incidence of amyloidosis in a series of greater than 50 necropsies on paraplegic patients. It would be unreasonable to make deductions on the incidence of amyloidosis from any smaller series.

Dalton *et al.* included the cases described by Dietrick and Russi (1958) and their incidence figures are as follows—

	Cases of Amyloidosis	Number of Post-mortems	Incidence %
Dietrick and Russi, 1958	12	55	23·5
Additional cases	14	34	—
Totals (Dalton *et al.*, 1965)	26	89	29·2

These authors commented that, if the 15 patients dying within one year and the 9 with short-term paraplegia due to tumours are excluded, the figure of 26/65 (40%) is more meaningful.

The paper of Nyquist and Bors (1967), mentioned before (p. 14), described 24 cases of amyloidosis in 99 necropsies (24·2%). Of these, 13 died in uraemia. For various reasons, including overlooking the diagnosis when the necropsy was performed for the Coroner, they thought their figures did not accurately reflect the incidence of secondary amyloidosis in paraplegia. They thought that the total incidence of amyloidosis in 1,851 traumatic myelopathy patients, living and dead, could be estimated at about 2 per cent.

The figures from these two papers agree fairly closely with the findings in this series, i.e.—

1963. 48 cases of amyloidosis in 122 chronic paraplegics (39%)
1965. 65 cases of amyloidosis in 174 chronic paraplegics (37%).

It seems that evidence of amyloidosis will be found in about 30–40 per cent of necropsies performed on chronic paraplegic patients.

DURING LIFE

All previous authors have produced estimates of the incidence of amyloidosis based upon post-mortem material of patients dying in hospital. The fallacies of such estimates for arriving at the true incidence of this condition among a living population of paraplegics are well recognised. The patients are selected by virtue of being in hospital, and are often war pensioners or older patients with no dependents either able or willing to look after them. Again, selection depends upon the particular outlook and interests of the clinicians attending the patients. The large American Units catering for war pensioners

naturally have a great predominance of male patients.

Where studies have been carried out on living patients, the diagnosis of amyloidosis has usually been made late in the condition, either when the patient is suffering from advanced renal failure or from the nephrotic syndrome.

After working at Stoke Mandeville Hospital for several years, where amyloidosis was often found at necropsy when it was not suspected during life, and stimulated by the paper of Arapakis and Tribe (1963), which suggested that rectal biopsy was an excellent screening method for amyloidosis, Dr Silver carried out a prospective study of the patients at the Liverpool Regional Paraplegic Centre to determine—

1. The incidence of amyloidosis in a representative cross-section of paraplegic patients
2. The prognosis of this condition
3. The early clinical manifestations.

Method

The method described by Arapakis and Tribe (1963) was followed. One or two specimens of rectal biopsy were taken with biopsy forceps and placed immediately into formal saline and then sent to two independent Pathologists, one of whom had been instructed by Dr Tribe in his staining methods, the other of whom was already carrying out routine biopsies for amyloidosis.

Material

Rectal biopsies were performed on 101 patients who were attending the Liverpool Regional Paraplegic Centre. The details are shown in Table 6.2. It is apparent that a high proportion of these patients were likely candidates for secondary amyloidosis.

Results

A total of 149 rectal biopsies on 101 patients were carried out. Biopsies were positive on two patients. Both died subsequently and at necropsy were found to have extensive amyloidosis of their kidneys.

A further two patients, both of whom had a picture of severe advanced amyloidosis, suggested by a nephrotic syndrome, had negative rectal biopsies during life, but at necropsy were found to have amyloidosis within their kidneys.

One additional patient, also with a nephrotic picture and a negative rectal biopsy, had a large stone removed with part of his kidney. He is still relatively well and back at work, but histological examination of the kidney revealed advanced amyloidosis. No patient from the rest of the series is known to have died.

TABLE 6.2
Rectal biopsy series (Liverpool Regional Paraplegic Centre, Southport)

SEX   96 males   5 females
AGE   Average age 43 years (range 16–68)
    Up to 30 years   18 cases
    31–40 years   19 cases
    41–50 years   39 cases
    51–60 years   16 cases
    Over 60 years   9 cases

SURVIVAL TIME SINCE PARAPLEGIA   Range 1–56 years
89 cases survived longer than four years with an average survival time of 12·5 years.

CAUSES OF PARAPLEGIA

    Traumatic or gunshot wound   71 cases
    Non-traumatic   30 cases

LEVELS OF PARAPLEGIA	COMPLETE	INCOMPLETE	TOTAL
Cervical	2	20	22
Thoracic 1–4	9	1	10
Thoracic 5–8	13	6	19
Thoracic 9–12	22	6	28
Lumbar and cauda equina	8	14	22

AETIOLOGICAL FACTORS	NO. OF CASES
Pressure sores	77
Pressure sores with osteomyelitis	49
Chronic urinary infection	94
Calculosis	8
Hydronephrosis	18

Comment

Although only 2 of the 101 patients had positive rectal biopsies; in this series, 5 are known to have had amyloidosis. These results, based on relatively small numbers, reflect on the accuracy of rectal biopsy as a means of diagnosing amyloidosis and this will be discussed later in connection with the pathological findings (p. 83). It is also difficult to make an accurate prediction concerning the incidence of amyloidosis, which must vary enormously with such factors as treatment, survival time and the incidence of septic complications. It does appear, however, that among paraplegic patients under review in Spinal Centres, up to 5 per cent of patients have amyloidosis.

Classification of Amyloidosis

All classifications of amyloidosis up to the present have been based on simple anatomical or clinico-pathological criteria. Symmers (1956) reviewed previous classifications and pointed out that 'a rational classification will not be possible until we know a great deal more than at present about the aetiology and pathogenesis of the various forms of amyloidosis and their relation to immunological response and metabolism of proteins and other substances'. At that time, he suggested the following classification, still the best for practical purposes—

1. *Generalised secondary amyloidosis.* Generalised amyloidosis associated with a recognised predisposing disease.
2. *Generalised primary amyloidosis.* Generalised amyloidosis in the absence of any recognised predisposing disease.
3. *Localised amyloidosis.*

More recently, Missmahl, working with various authors in Israel (Missmahl and Gafni, 1963; Heller *et al.*, 1964), has differentiated cases of generalised amyloidosis into two groups, based on a histological study of sections stained by Congo Red and examined with the polarising microscope. They have termed these groups peri-reticulin and peri-collagen.

All cases of amyloidosis associated with the septic complications of paraplegia fall into the generalised secondary amyloidosis and perireticulin groups, and have a 'typical' anatomical distribution (King, 1948). Until a more definite histochemical distinction is possible, these anatomical clinico-pathological terms provide only a crude way of classifying cases of generalised amyloidosis. They fail to take into account the wide diversity of distribution between individual cases, and an additional anatomical division into vascular and parenchymal types has been suggested by the author (Tribe, 1966) and is discussed later in this chapter.

Finding in the Present Series

In 174 necropsies performed on patients with chronic paraplegia, 65 cases of amyloidosis were found. No cases were found among the acute paraplegics, and no cases were included without histological proof. Some essential details of these cases are presented in Table 6.3.

AETIOLOGICAL FACTORS

The two most important complications of paraplegia are pressure sores and urinary tract infection. These may lead to death directly, or indirectly, as the predisposing causes of amyloidosis.

Previous literature (Table 6.1) suggested that decubitus ulceration, often with underlying osteo-myelitis, is the chief factor in producing amyloidosis in paraplegia. For this reason, the incidence of pressure sores and osteomyelitis was studied in these patients. The sites and severity of pressure sores were well recorded in the clinical notes, but the true incidence of underlying osteomyelitis was not so easy to assess. Only those cases in which either radio-logical or operative evidence of bone suppuration

TABLE 6.3

Amyloidosis in chronic paraplegia (65 cases)

DISTRIBUTION

Group	No. of cases	No. of cases with amyloidosis	Percentage
Group A. Traumatic paraplegia Death related to paraplegia	97	51	53
Group B. Traumatic paraplegia Death unrelated to paraplegia	26	4*	15
Group C. Non-traumatic paraplegia Death related to paraplegia	20	8	40
Group D. Non-traumatic paraplegia Death unrelated to paraplegia	31	2†	6

The remaining 63 cases were all associated with chronic infection occurring as a direct complication of paraplegia.

AGE   Average age at death was 39·9 years.

Up to 30 years	8 cases
31–40 years	27 cases
41–50 years	17 cases
51–60 years	9 cases
Over 60 years	4 cases

LEVELS OF PARAPLEGIA	COMPLETE	INCOMPLETE	TOTAL
Cervical	6	8	14
Thoracic 1–4	5	0	5
Thoracic 5–8	15	0	15
Thoracic 9–12	20	1	21
Lumbar and cauda equina	3	6	9
Not recorded	1	0	1

SURVIVAL TIMES SINCE ONSET OF PARAPLEGIA

The average survival time of 63 cases was 11·8 years from the onset of paraplegia.
The shortest survival time in 63 cases was 1·5 years from the onset of paraplegia.‡
The longest survival time in 63 cases was 25 years from the onset of paraplegia.

---

* One of these cases had pulmonary tuberculosis.
† One of these cases had metastatic neuroblastoma.
‡ This case died with amyloid disease only 7 months after the onset of pressure sores (*see* p. 74).

was found in life have been included. Only 5 of the 65 patients with amyloidosis had no clinically recorded pressure sores, and in only 18 patients was there no evidence of osteomyelitis.

Both clinical and pathological evidence was used in judging the part played by urinary tract sepsis in the causation of amyloidosis. All cases had long-standing urinary infection and 42 had suprapubic cystotomies at some time. At necropsy, 28 cases showed unilateral or bilateral pyonephrosis, and of the 61 cases in which kidney tissue was available for microscopy, only 4 showed no evidence of pyelonephritis. Calculosis of the upper urinary tract had been present during life in 23 cases, and was found at necropsy in 15 cases.

These aetiological factors are represented as percentages in Table 6.4.

TABLE 6.4

Aetiological factors in 65 cases of amyloidosis and chronic paraplegia

Aetiological factors	No. of cases	Percentage
Pressure sores	60	92
Pressure sores with radiological and/or operative evidence of underlying osteomyelitis	47	72
Chronic urinary infection	65	100
Chronic pyelonephritis	61	94
Suprapubic cystotomy during life	42	65
Pyonephrosis at post-mortem	28	43
Calculosis in life	23	35
Calculosis at necropsy	15	23

In this series, amyloidosis was usually due to a combination of chronic pressure sores, frequently associated with underlying osteomyelitis, and chronic urinary tract suppuration sometimes aggravated by calculosis. This series does show, however, that amyloidosis may occur in paraplegics without pressure sores, and in these cases the amyloidosis presumably resulted solely from chronic urinary tract infection. This has not been reported by other authors, and a brief case-history of one of these patients is now presented to support our view.

Case History

G. A. aged fifty-six at the time of his death, suffered an incomplete traumatic paraplegia at L.3 from a mining accident at the age of forty. He was first admitted to Stoke Mandeville Hospital when aged forty-three with a chronic urinary infection and bilateral hydronephrosis.

At this time he had had no significant pressure sores since his accident, and did not develop any during the remainder of his life.

His urinary infection persisted and four years later, aged forty-seven, he became hypertensive (his blood pressure remaining between 150/110 and 220/150 for the rest of his life). This was associated with slowly deteriorating renal function, and six months before his death his blood urea was 110 mg per cent, with a urea clearance of 10 per cent and gross proteinuria. Prior to death, a rectal biopsy was suggestive of amyloidosis and his blood urea reached 500 mg per cent.

At necropsy, the heart was moderately enlarged from left ventricular hypertrophy with only mild coronary atheroma. The kidneys showed a mild chronic bilateral pyonephrosis with gross scarring and reduction in thickness of the surviving renal tissue. Microscopy revealed widespread generalised amyloidosis (Grade 111) involving the following organs: thyroid + +, heart ±, liver + +, spleen + + +, adrenals +, pancreas +, kidneys + + +, stomach + +, intestines +, and rectum ±. The kidneys showed widespread focal atrophic chronic pyelonephritis with evidence of recent and old pelvi-calyceal infection, and all the surviving glomeruli were completely filled with amyloid material. There was no evidence of malignant hypertension.

The final cause of death in this case was considered to be renal failure from a combination of chronic pyelonephritis, pyonephroses, and amyloidosis with hypertensive heart disease probably secondary to chronic renal disease. In this case, the amyloidosis was thought to be solely due to chronic renal suppuration.

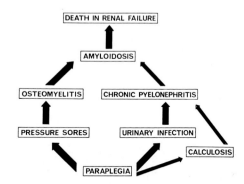

FIG. 6.1. Aetiology of amyloidosis in chronic paraplegia.

This series also shows that in some cases amyloidosis occurs predominantly from pressure sores and osteomyelitis with only minimal urinary tract sepsis, restricted to the bladder. These findings are summarised in Fig. 6.1.

From a study of all the chronic paraplegics in this series, a fair generalisation can be made that the greater the number and severity of septic complications the greater the chance of developing secondary amyloidosis. It is apparent, however, that in assessing any individual case this generalisation may prove incorrect.

Several patients had persistent pressure sores, with chronic sinuses and osteomyelitis, together with chronic renal sepsis, yet at necropsy showed no evidence of amyloidosis. In contrast, there were a few patients in whom pressure sores occurred early in their lives as paraplegics, and which were quickly healed with no recurrence. However, in spite of only mild subsequent renal sepsis, post-mortem examination of these patients many years later revealed widespread severe amyloidosis.

It was thought that a susceptibility to amyloidosis might be related to the level of the paraplegia, and Table 6.5 shows that there was a higher percentage of cases among the chronic quadriplegic patients, but that the incidence among the thoracic and lumbar groups was fairly constant.

TABLE 6.5

Amyloidosis and chronic paraplegia
(Incidence in relation to level of spinal lesion)

Level of spinal lesion	Total no. of patients	Patients with amyloidosis	Percentage
Cervical	28	13	46·5
Thoracic 1–4	15	5	33
Thoracic 5–8	39	14	36
Thoracic 9–12	63	21	33
Lumbar and cauda equina	26	9	34·5
Totals	171*	62†	

* Three patients with levels of injury unrecorded not included.

† Two cases unrelated to septic complications of paraplegia, and one patient with level of injury unrecorded, not included.

It seems likely that the quadriplegic, whose prognosis is more precarious, is more likely to develop amyloidosis from sepsis rather than to any specific relationship to the level or degree of paralysis itself. Only further analysis of a greater number of cases will confirm this. There is much to be learnt before the aetiology of secondary amyloidosis in chronic paraplegia is fully understood.

Clinical and Laboratory Findings

INTRODUCTION

At the National Spinal Injuries Centre, Stoke Mandeville Hospital, 11 paraplegic patients who had systemic amyloidosis were described by Doggart *et al.* in 1966. These 11, together with the 5 patients found in the rectal biopsy series at the Liverpool Regional Paraplegic Centre (described earlier), have been studied and the total 16 patients illustrate the clinical and laboratory findings during life in amyloidosis secondary to chronic paraplegia. Their details are given in the large Table 6.6.

The 16 patients were all male and their ages ranged between twenty-seven and fifty-nine years. Twelve patients were paralysed as a result of trauma, and there was one example each of multiple sclerosis, extradural abscess, haemangioma, and neuromyelitis optica. It has already been shown that traumatic paraplegics carry no more risk of developing amyloidosis than paraplegics paralysed from other causes. The high proportion of traumatic paraplegics in this and the post-mortem series merely reflects the precedence that is given, both at the National Spinal Injury Centre and at the Liverpool Regional Paraplegic Centre, to the admission of traumatic cases.

CLINICAL MANIFESTATIONS

Oedema is the most striking clinical manifestation of amyloidosis in paraplegic patients. This is widespread and particularly obvious around the face. It was present in 8 of the 11 patients examined in 1966 (Doggart *et al.*) and in all the patients where the 24-hour urinary protein excretion was measured (7 of the 8) it was above 4·9 G. This is in keeping with the findings of Milne (1962), who stated that in generalised amyloidosis, 50 per cent of the patients will develop oedema at some stage, and that oedema will not be present unless more than 5 G of protein are lost in the urine each day. Brod (1962) also found oedema in 45 per cent of his cases. The protein loss in the urine was above 5 G a day in 90 per cent of his cases. Oedema is not invariably present, and may well be overlooked or its significance not appreciated, since many paraplegics suffer from postural oedema of their lower limbs from their lack of mobility and prolonged recumbency which impairs the venous return from the lower limbs. A further important cause of oedema in the lower limbs of paraplegic patients occurs during the acute phase, when many paraplegic patients have significant deep vein thrombosis of their lower limbs. This is most suggestive when there is a history of a swollen hot leg, but it is well recognised that deep vein thrombosis often occurs with no clinical signs or symptoms. In 1954,

Bors found that of 99 patients 58 had evidence of venous occlusion, and in 1963 Phillips found that of 25 paraplegic patients 6 had evidence of deep vein thrombosis.

Tetraplegic patients are also liable to develop swelling of their hands, but this occurs as early as six weeks after injury when they are first beginning to sit up. This is frequently associated with swelling and deformity of the joints of the hands.

Haemorrhage

Many patients with amyloidosis suffer from re-current small haemorrhages from the mucous membranes. This has been recognised for some time, though very little has been written on the subject, apart from Comarr (1958) and Malament (1963) who suggested that the bleeding was due to amyloid infiltration of the blood vessels. This phenomenon was looked for in the 5 patients seen in Southport and was present in 4 cases.

Illustrative Cases

1. C. K., during the last six months of his life, suffered many small recurrent nose bleeds. They were not true heavy epistaxes. On two occasions he had smoky dark red urine. There were no clots but it was a similar type of bleeding to that seen after decompression of a distended bladder. On neither of these occasions had there been a preceding blocked catheter or retention of urine.

2. J. C., on six different occasions during the last twelve months of his life, suffered recurrent haemorrhages from his bladder which was small and contracted. On one occasion the haemorrhage was so severe that he had to be admitted to hospital. Each time the haemorrhage occurred it was at least seven days after his catheter had been changed and this suggests that no trauma was involved. On one occasion the haemorrhage was so severe that a cystoscopy was performed, and this showed that he had multiple granulations of the bladder, biopsy of which showed inflammatory tissue. On one admission to hospital he had a sub-conjunctival haemorrhage which persisted for about ten days and then gradually subsided. At necropsy bleeding from the mucous membrane of his mouth and gums appeared to be a terminal event.

3. E. D. was admitted on two occasions, during his last year of life, with severe haematuria which subsided with symptomatic treatment. He had recurrent heavy epistaxes which were so severe that he required adrena-line packs to stop the bleeding. He was severely hyper-tensive with a blood pressure of 260/140.

4. J. R. was admitted terminally with a history of a bladder haemorrhage. On admission he had dark smoky urine with old altered blood, but no clots.

There are many possible causes of this bleeding—

1. Anaemia.
2. Deficiency of fibrinogen.

3. Deficiency of vitamin C.
4. Infiltration of the blood vessels with amyloid (suggested by Malament and found by Missen and Tribe, 1968) in amyloidosis associated with rheumatoid arthritis (*see* p. 84).
5. Raised blood pressure.
6. Raised blood urea (a bleeding tendency is well recognised in acute renal failure due to quanti-tative and qualitative defects in platelets).
7. Multiple deficiencies of vitamins and proteins.

It is of interest that in primary macroglobulinaemia (Waldenström), where there is an abnormality of the plasma proteins, particularly of the globulin fraction, one of the most striking features is a general haemor-rhagic tendency with bleeding from the nose and gums. The possible relationship of this bleeding to amyloidosis would provide an interesting field for further research.

Toxaemia

Four of the patients from the post-mortem series of Tribe, and one from Southport, died of acute bacterial endocarditis. Of these, 4 had widespread amyloidosis. With modern antibiotics it is unusual, both in paraplegia and in general medicine, for such cases to be seen, and it is possible that the toxaemia was associated with amyloidosis. It seems likely that the widespread infiltration of amyloid material, with involvement of bone marrow, lymph glands, gut, liver, spleen, and other reticulo-endothelial organs impedes the defence mechanisms of the body with consequent susceptibility to overwhelming sepsis.

There was no evidence that amyloidosis prevented pressure sores from healing, or interfered with the primary healing of surgical wounds. Many patients had severe pressure sores, with underlying osteo-myelitis, most frequently around the hip. The treat-ment of these sores is particularly difficult since flexor spasms result in movements of the hip with shearing stresses that allow pus to pocket and penetrate around the tissue planes. These sores were probably the initial cause of the amyloidosis, and their failure to heal was due to local anatomical factors and not to the systemic amyloidosis. How-ever, where superficial sores occurred or where the osteomyelitis was not of great severity, no apparent difference in the rate of healing was noted. Many of these patients were admitted with severe sores and these healed even though amyloidosis was known to be present.

Illustrative Cases

1. C. K., who was paralysed below T.10 as the result of an accident, developed a brain tumour that necessitated his transfer to other hospitals for specialised treatment.

Name	Age at time of study	Lesion	Status	Duration of injury or illness (in years)	Relevant history
H.M.	48	C6 Trauma	Dead 1 year after + rectal biopsy	13	Injury at 35. Severe pressure sores with osteomyelitis. Automati micturition for next 12 years with normal IVP but persistent infectior Epileptic fits at 47. Admitted at 48 with blood urea of 54 mg/100 m rising to 175 mg/100 ml. Normotensive. Died at home.
G.W.	59 (died 62)	T2 Trauma	Dead 3 years after + rectal biopsy	9	Injured at 53. Persistent urinary infection but normal IVP. Pressur sores with osteomyelitis. Oedematous: serum albumin 1·9 G/100 m serum globulin 3·7 G/100 ml. Proteinuria 4·9 G/24 hr. Normotensive
K.W.	32 (now 35)	T6 Trauma	Alive 3 years after + rectal biopsy	15	Injured at 20. Immediate suprapubic cystotomy. Vesical stones Pressure sores with osteomyelitis. Serum albumin 3·2 G/100 ml, serun globulin 4·1 G/100 ml. Proteinuria 7·5 G/24 hr.
M.F.	32	T7 Trauma	Dead 1 year after + rectal biopsy	6	Injured at 26. Pressure sores with osteomyelitis. Automatic micturi tion. At 31, oedematous: Serum albumin 0·9 G/100 ml, serum globuli 2·0 G/100 ml. Proteinuria 12·8 G/24 hr. Positive Congo Red test Died after subarachnoid haemorrhage. Amyloidosis confirmed a post-mortem.
P.R.	31	T7 Trauma	Dead	10	Injured at 21. Automatic micturition, At 26, hydronephrosis left, n secretion on right; bilateral reflux; diverticula of bladder. At 31 hypertensive retinopathy. Post-mortem diagnosis of renal amyloidosis
G.M.	27 (now 31)	T10 Trauma	Alive 4 years after + rectal biopsy	12½	Injured at 19. Pressure sores with osteomyelitis and a periurethra abscess. Suprapubic cystotomy performed. Hydronephrosis, hydro ureter and diverticula. Oedematous: serum globulin 2·4 G/100 m serum albumin 0·4 G/100 ml. Serum cholesterol 450 mg/100 m Proteinuria 13·6 G/24 hr.
P.O'D.	48 (now 52)	T11 Haemangioma	Alive 4 years after + rectal biopsy	10	Haemangioma of cord at 42. Pressure sores with osteomyelitis. Dis charged at 45 with automatic bladder, sterile urine and bilatera hydronephrosis. At 48, BP 150/100. Proteinuria 2·0 G/24 hr.
W.C.	56	T12 Trauma	Dead	19	Injured at 37. Immediate suprapubic cystotomy. Infected urine. A 46, BP 175/110. At 52, nephrectomy for renal calculus; at 53, pressur sores; serum albumin 3·6 G/100 ml, serum globulin 3·7 G/100 m At 54, proteinuria 2·8 G/24 hr. Admitted terminally, confused an oliguric. Post-mortem amyloidosis.
G.A.	55	L3 Trauma	Dead + rectal biopsy	15	Injured at 40. Pressure sores. Dribbling incontinence of urine. At 4 hydronephrosis. BP 220/150; at 45, indwelling catheter. Died at 5 chronic pyelonephritis and renal amyloidosis.
W.B.	43	Multiple sclerosis	Dead 1 year after + rectal biopsy	20	Diagnosed as multiple sclerosis at 23. Unable to walk by 38. At 3 sores causing osteomyelitis. IVP showed vesical calculus; serur albumin 2·1 G/100 ml, serum globulin 3·4 G/100 ml.
T.H.	41	T12 Trauma	Alive 3 years after + rectal biopsy	5	Admitted within 10 days of injury, urine rendered sterile; discharge with blood urea 41 mg/100 ml 252 days after injury. Re-admitted 15 days later with residual of 20 oz little secretion on IVP. Infected urine proteinuria; treated by tidal drainage.
V.W.	34	T4 Trauma	Alive 6 months after − rectal biopsy. Op for calculus	14	Injured at 20. Extensive sores from outset, with urinary infection an suprapubic cystotomy. This was closed. Progressive hydronephros from 3 years after injury. Partially relieved by bladder neck operation Found to have a left sided calculus. Negative rectal biopsy. Amyloi found in the operation specimen.
E.D.	39	Neuromye-litis optica	Dead − rectal biopsy	13	Became ill at 27. Developed total paralysis below T4. Severe pressur sores for many years. Became hypertensive 9 years after onset. He ha reflux severe urinary infection and became oedematous. Repeate admissions with haematuria. Negative biopsy.
J.C.	48	T4 Trauma	Dead 3 years after + rectal biopsy	21	Injured at 27. Suprapubic cystotomy. Extensive bed sores. Righ nephrectomy at 28 for pyonephrosis. Normal IVP subsequently Became oedematous at 44. Rectal biopsy +. Put on steroids at 4 Poor function on IVP. Developed carcinoma of the penis an repeated episodes of haematuria.
J.R.	50	T10 Extradural abscess	Dead − rectal biopsy + renal biopsy	19	Staphylococcal abscess diagnosed at laminectomy. Sinuses an pressure sores. 38 hydronephrosis. 39 developed pulmonary TB. 4 BP 206/130. Developed extensive sores. 49 became oedematous Developed Wernicke encephalopathy. Died. Acute ulcerativ endocarditis.
C.K.	46	T10 Trauma	Dead 1 year after + rectal biopsy	20	Injured at 26. Multiple sores. Indwelling catheter. Stone in righ kidney. Reflux to right at 39 years. Brain tumour. Surgery and radic therapy. Enormous sores. Blood urea 88. Haematuria. Sores heale Died of brain tumour.

dema	BP	Intravenous pyelogram (IVP)	Urinary 24-hour protein (G/24 hr)	Plasma protein (G/100 ml)	Creatinine Serum (mg/100 ml)	Clearance (ml/min)	Urea Serum (mg/100 ml)	Clearance (% of average normal function)	Concentrating ability (mOs)
—	120/80 — 135/95	Normal—diverticula, no reflux	—	—	3·6 / 2·9	6 / 7	144 / 103	8 / 12	
es	110/80 — 140/90	Normal	4·9	Alb. 1·9–2·0 Glob. 3·6–5·9	0·8 / 0·7	69 / 79	31	44	552
—	150/90	Bladder stones	7·5	Alb. 3·2 Glob. 4·1	0·8 / 0·7	34 / 65	30 / 29	33 / 26	459
es	140/80 Progressing to 170/110	No function right kidney	12·8	Alb. 0·9 Glob. 2·0	3·8	19	99	—	
—	120/90 Hypertensive	Hydronephrosis on left, no secretion on the right	—	—	5·2 / 4·9 / 9·3 / 10·1	10 / 8 / 2 / 2	67 / 70 / 109 / 156	11 / 12 / 8 / 4	
es	130/90	Hydronephrosis, hydroureter, diverticula	13·6	Alb. 0·4 Glob. 2·4	0·7 / 0·8 / 0·7	86 / 65 / 73	30 / 29 / 38	— / — / 34	528
—	150/100	Bilateral hydronephrosis reflux	2·0	Alb. 3·2 Glob. 3·0	2·8 / 2·9	15 / 23	99 / 66	11 / 20	
—	175/110	Poor secretion	2·8	Alb. 3·6 Glob. 3·7	6·8	3	100		
—	220/150	Hydronephrosis	—	Alb. 3·9 Glob. 3·1	5·1	11	90	10	
—	180/120	Bladder stones	Less than 1·0	Alb. 2·1 Glob. 3·3	0·5 / 0·4	81 / 72	24 / 18	77 / —	577
—	—	Diverticula reflux, little secretion	—	Alb. 2·0 Glob. 5·3	1·7 / 1·3 / 2·0 / 1·7	44 / 67 / 50 / 56	81 / 36 / 46 / 62	24 / 44 / — / 29	
es	190/105	Progressive hydronephrosis, bilateral with left sided stone	14·0	Alb. 3·4 Glob. 5·1	2·2	25	45		
es	260/140	Poor demonstration, drip IVP	8·8	Alb. 3·4 Glob. 2·5	2·0 / 3·4	19 / 2·5	38		
es	100/70 160/90 160/100 After steroids	Poor function, drip IVP no demonstration	12–14	Alb. 2·8 Glob. 1·2			40 / 60 / 80 / 280		
es	206/130 130/90	Poor demonstration, drip IVP	20·0	Alb. 2·6 Glob. 1·7	3·7	18·5	52		
es	120/75	Stone right kidney	—	Alb. 3·4 Glob. 2·7	3·8		88		

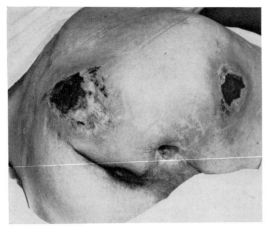

FIG. 6.2(*a*)

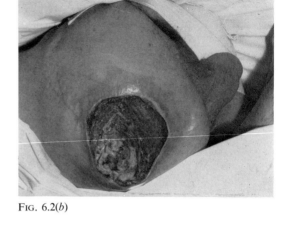

FIG. 6.2(*b*)

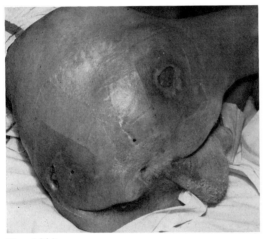

FIG. 6.2(*c*)

FIG. 6.2. (*a*) and (*b*) Illustrative case C.K. Extensive pressure sores on re-admission to Spinal Centre. At this time amyloidosis was diagnosed by rectal biopsy. (*c*) Following several months of regular turning, blood transfusions, and skin grafts the pressure sores have almost completely healed.

On departure from the Spinal Centre he had no pressure sores. When he returned to the Centre following treatment, he had large, deep and extensive sores (*see* Fig. 6.2). Amyloidosis was diagnosed by rectal biopsy (and subsequently confirmed at necropsy), but after extensive treatment, debridement, blood transfusion, skin grafting, etc., all the sores healed and he was allowed out of bed until he died some months later from a recurrence of his brain tumour.

2. J. C. had his little toe and metatarsal amputated for underlying osteomyelitis. The wound healed perfectly by first intention.

3. V. W. had a hemi-nephrectomy performed for a stone in his kidney. The loin scar healed perfectly by first intention and the patient is back at full time work.

4. W. B. was admitted to Stoke Mandeville Hospital with extensive pressure sores. After some months of treatment all these sores were healed despite his amyloidosis.

Laboratory Findings

PROTEINURIA

The significance of proteinuria in a single specimen of urine from a paraplegic patient is difficult to assess. A specimen of urine is usually tested with Clinistix and this provides only a rough guide to the amount of protein present. The majority of paraplegic patients have a low grade infection of their urinary tract; 94 of 101 patients in the Southport biopsy series had a urinary infection. If this involves the kidney and causes chronic pyelonephritis, 'the pathological process in the neighbourhood of the glomeruli causes proteinuria, perhaps due to an interference with the blood supply, allowing for an increased diffusion of plasma proteins into the glomerular filtrate' (Brod, 1962). In addition, chronic cystitis and low grade urethritis, both of which are common in paraplegic patients, can produce proteinuria. However, in these conditions the loss of protein is unlikely to be greater than 5 G a day, and will not *per se* cause systemic disturbance as the result of hypoproteinaemia.

To determine the significance of proteinuria, estimations must be made on 24-hour urine samples. As was shown before, all the patients with amyloidosis who were oedematous lost more than 4·9 G of protein in twenty-four hours. In the 3 patients with amyloid without oedema, the protein lost was less than 3 G in a 24-hour urine sample. Many of the 101 patients who had rectal biopsies at Southport, had proteinuria on routine urine testing with Clinistix. In 12 of these, the 24-hour protein loss was estimated; the figures ranged between 0·75–6 G in twenty-four hours.

There is an overlap in these findings with the patients from the amyloid group. In view of the negative rectal biopsies in 3 of the patients, who were subsequently found to have renal amyloidosis, the finding of a protein loss in the urine of above 5 G a day is strongly suggestive of renal amyloidosis but a lower figure does not exclude this condition.

This is confirmed by Arapakis and Tribe (1963) who found proteinuria in only 3 of their 6 patients with positive rectal biopsies for amyloidosis.

HYPOPROTEINAEMIA

Since the work of Robinson in 1954, a special interest has been taken at Stoke Mandeville in the plasma albumin and globulin levels in paraplegic patients. There are many factors which influence the level of plasma proteins. Initially, immediately after cord injury, there is a fall in the albumin and a rise in the globulin. Subsequently, when the acute injury has subsided, there is a gradual return to near normal levels. This return to normal will be delayed by any infection and the most frequent cause is protein loss from unhealed pressure sores.

PLASMA ALBUMIN

In the paraplegic patient with no pressure sores, the kidneys play the chief part in altering the level of plasma albumin. Albuminuria is well recognised as being the earliest clinical sign of renal amyloidosis (Loughbridge, 1960) and, terminally, these patients show a classical nephrotic syndrome. Patients with amyloid may lose up to 20 G of protein a day in their urine. Electrophoresis reveals that this protein is almost entirely albumin. The severe albuminuria is reflected in the plasma albumin levels.

Table 6.7 shows the lowest recorded plasma albumin levels in the 65 post-mortem cases of amyloidosis in chronic paraplegia (Tribe).

TABLE 6.7

Plasma albumin levels in chronic paraplegics with amyloidosis

Less than 1·0 G/100 ml	8 cases (0·3, 0·4, 0·45, 0·5, 0·5, 0·8, 0·8, and 0·9)
1·0–2·0 G/100 ml	20 cases
2·0–3·0 G/100 ml	18 cases
More than 3·0 G/100 ml	1 case
Not recorded	18 cases

The relationship of the serum albumin to the urinary loss of albumin is given in Table 6.6, which shows that the lowest levels tend to be found in those patients with the highest loss in the urine: though it should not be forgotten that these patients might well be losing even more protein from chronic discharging sinuses or pressure sores. There are other factors that regulate the serum albumin level, such as the level of nutrition of the patient, blood transfusions, a high protein diet, treatment of the underlying infections, and the use of steroids. Many patients were initially admitted with low serum albumin levels as the result of amyloidosis and pressure sores, and these could be temporarily restored to normal by high protein diet and blood transfusions.

RENAL FUNCTION TESTS

The serum levels, and clearances, of creatinine and urea were estimated in the majority of patients in the Southport series. A limited number of tests to find the concentrating ability of the kidneys were performed by depriving the patient of fluid overnight and then measuring the maximum concentration of the urine the next morning with an advanced osmometer. The results of these tests are shown in Table 6.6. It was hoped that these tests might differentiate renal conditions, since on pathological grounds it could be postulated that there would be predominantly glomerular involvement with preservation of tubular function in pure renal amyloidosis and the converse in pyelonephritis. This proved incorrect and the tests did not distinguish between pure renal amyloidosis, renal amyloidosis with chronic pyelonephritis, and chronic pyelonephritis. This is hardly surprising in view of the frequent coexistence of amyloidosis and chronic pyelonephritis at necropsy. The diagnosis of renal amyloidosis was suspected when there was heavy proteinuria (above 5 G a day) and established by a positive biopsy.

Renal function tests did prove of value in assessing the prognosis of these patients. The finding of a low endogenous creatinine clearance (below 20 ml/min) carried a poor prognosis and, of the 9 patients who died, only 2 had clearances above 20 ml/min. In contrast, none of the 5 patients who are still alive had clearances below 20 ml/min. This confirms Metcoff's view (1962) that 'glomerular filtration rates progressively lowered to less than 30 per cent of normal after one to two years of the active nephrotic syndrome have an ominous significance'.

Urea clearances were carried out in only 9 patients in the Southport series, as they did not give as reproducible and as consistent results as the creatinine clearance. Nevertheless, when the urea clearances were below 20 per cent of the average normal (in 4 of the 9 patients), there was a close correlation between the creatinine and the urea clearances and the prognosis, and 3 of the 4 patients are now dead. This correlation did not hold at higher values.

High serum levels of creatinine were a reliable indication of impaired renal function, since in the 15 patients where it was estimated those patients (8) with values above 3 mg/100 ml are now dead. In contrast, 5 of the 7 patients who had values below 3 mg/100 ml are still alive. A limited number of urea clearances, serum creatinine, and creatinine clearances, were performed during life on the patients in the post-mortem series (Tribe), and the results of these tests confirm those found in the Southport series described above.

The blood urea was the most frequently performed test of renal function, and serial estimations were carried out in all patients both at Southport and Stoke Mandeville. It proved to be an unreliable

estimate of renal function unless the patient was in terminal renal failure. Table 6.8 gives the figures of the terminal blood ureas from the 65 post-mortem cases.

TABLE 6.8

Terminal blood urea levels (i.e. within one week of death) in 65 post-mortem cases of Amyloidosis in Chronic Paraplegia (Tribe)

	NO. OF CASES
Normal	6
40–100 mg%	3
100–200 mg%	14
200–300 mg%	14
Greater than 300 mg%	22
Not recorded	6

The value of renal function tests in paraplegic patients has been discussed earlier in this book (p. 30). It is recognised, following the work of Berlyne *et al.* (1964), that the endogenous creatinine clearance does not give an accurate indication of the glomerular filtration rate when compared with the inulin clearance and that the serum levels of creatinine do not rise until renal failure is well advanced. The disadvantages of blood urea estimations need little stressing, since it fluctuates with many factors apart from the renal function of the patients. Further research, using more accurate clearance techniques coupled with biopsy studies, will yield much more information about the influence of renal amyloidosis upon renal function.

Methods of Diagnosing Amyloidosis in Life

CONGO RED TEST

This test, introduced by Bennhold in 1923, has remained the only routine biochemical test for the diagnosis of amyloidosis. Its value is marred by the large number of false negative results (Stemmerman and Auerbach, 1944; Blum and Sohar, 1962), and as means of diagnosing amyloidosis in life it has now been replaced by tissue biopsy.

Congo Red tests have not been employed at Stoke Mandeville Hospital for some years, due to toxic reactions, and only 11 tests had been performed on these 65 cases during life. The results were—

		No. of cases	Degree of amyloidosis at necropsy	
Positive	10% dye retained after 1 hour	4	2 severe	2 moderate
Suggestive	10–40% dye retained after 1 hour	3	1 severe	2 moderate
Negative	40% dye retained after 1 hour	4	2 moderate	2 slight

All these tests were performed within two years of death and, as can be seen, the degree of Congo Red retention was roughly related to the severity of the amyloidosis found at post-mortem. However, as a means of definite diagnosis during life these tests had only limited value.

BIOPSY METHODS

Certain sites are now well recognised as suitable for the biopsy diagnosis of amyloidosis, namely, gingiva, liver, kidney, and rectum. Other sites such as lymph nodes, upper intestinal tract, and bone marrow have been tried in small groups of cases, but their value is as yet uncertain. Tribe (1966) reviewed these methods and assessed their value from post-mortem material in cases of secondary amyloidosis occurring in patients with chronic arthritis and chronic paraplegia. Certain points are worth accentuating.

Several authors have advocated rectal biopsy as the best method of diagnosing amyloidosis (Ducrot *et al.*, 1961; Fentem *et al.*, 1963; Blum and Sohar, 1962; Arapakis and Tribe, 1963). However, it should be appreciated that rectal biopsy is not infallible; Blum and Sohar obtained 47 positive results in 62 known cases (75%) of generalised amyloidosis, and Tribe (1966) thought 90 per cent accuracy should be obtainable in generalised secondary amyloidosis. Therefore, if the rectal biopsy is negative and the clinical and laboratory findings are strongly suggestive of amyloidosis, biopsy of the upper gastro-intestinal tract by means of a Crosby capsule is suggested on pathological grounds (*see* p. 82) before attempting a renal biopsy which still has intrinsic dangers.

It should also be stressed that any tissue removed by the surgeons from chronic paraplegics should be routinely stained for amyloid. A case quoted before (Tribe, 1966) illustrates this.

A man, now aged forty-six, had complete paraplegia at T.10 in 1954. This was followed by severe pressure sores with underlying osteomyelitis, and a persistent urinary infection. By the summer of 1964, he was in early renal failure with signs of a nephrotic syndrome; however, a rectal biopsy showed no amyloid. In January 1965, he had a cholecystectomy for biliary colic and appendicectomy. Extensive amyloid infiltration was found throughout the stroma of the mucosa of the gall bladder and very early desposition in some of the arterioles in the submucosa of the appendix.

Pathological Findings

MACROSCOPIC

The naked-eye diagnosis of amyloidosis was only rarely made with confidence in this series, and no cases were included without histochemical confirmation. Several cases thought to be amyloidosis at necropsy showed no histological evidence of this disease, and several cases with no naked-eye changes suggestive of amyloidosis showed widespread amyloid deposition on microscopy. For this reason, several patients who died between 1945 and 1950 and showed changes suggestive of amyloidosis at necropsy have been excluded since there was no material available for retrospective histological study.

Only four organs, liver, spleen, kidneys, and adrenals, showed macroscopic evidence of amyloidosis and the naked-eye changes in these organs will now be described.

Liver

One of the features in this series was the rarity of severe amyloid disease of the liver. Liver weights were available in 61 cases—

Under 40 oz	3 cases	Less than normal 14
40–50 oz	11 cases	
51–60 oz	17 cases	Within normal range 17
61–70 oz	10 cases	Greater than normal 30
71–80 oz	7 cases	
Greater than 80 oz	13 cases	

In a few cases, the liver had the characteristic enlarged, firm waxy appearance of secondary amyloidosis. More often the appearances were quite non-specific. In one patient who died shortly after a Congo Red test, the liver, spleen, and kidneys had a striking pink hue.

The iodine test was applied to the liver in many cases, and a poor correlation was obtained with the final histological findings. It is thought that this crude test, performed at the time of post-mortem examination, should be abandoned since, in those few cases in which one obtains a true 'mahogany' brown staining, the general appearance and feel of the liver is quite characteristic.

Spleen

Enlargement of the spleen was found more frequently than enlargement of either the liver or kidneys, and in the absence of other causes of splenomegaly, was suggestive of amyloidosis. Splenic weights were available in 61 cases—

Up to 5 oz	6 cases	Less than normal 6
5–6 oz	7 cases	Within normal range 7
7–8 oz	14 cases	
9–11 oz	17 cases	
12–15 oz	9 cases	Greater than normal 48
15–20 oz	5 cases	
Greater than 20 oz	3 cases	
(26 oz, 28 oz, and 32 oz)		

The enlargement of the spleen was not often marked and, since it is recognised that the spleen must be at least twice normal size before it is palpable, in only 17 of the 61 cases with splenic weights available (28%) might the spleen have been felt on clinical examination. The classical 'sago' spleen was occasionally seen, but more often it was enlarged with a firm waxy pink homogeneous cut surface.

Kidney

The diagnosis of amyloidosis from the naked-eye appearances of the kidneys was only possible in the few cases of 'pure' renal amyloidosis. Here, the

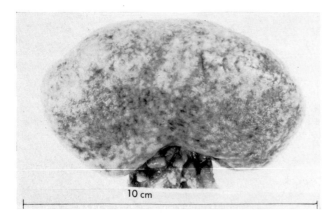

FIG. 6.3. External subcapsular appearance of a kidney from a sixty-one year old paraplegic who died in renal failure from 'pure renal amyloidosis'. The kidney surface shows a fine granularity with no gross scarring.

kidneys were enlarged, the capsules stripped easily revealing finely nodular surfaces with no gross scarring (Fig. 6.3). On section, the cortical tissue was thickened without gross alteration of the renal architecture, although the cortico-medullary margins were usually blurred. The renal tissue had a characteristic pale, firm, white waxy glistening appearance (Fig. 6.4). In one case a horseshoe kidney had this characteristic appearance (Fig. 6.5).

There was another small group of enlarged kidneys which showed a few small deep subcortical scars of focal pyelonephritis (Figs. 6.6 and 6.7). On section this group showed a similar pale waxy renal tissue and there was frequently a terminal active pyonephrosis (Fig. 6.8).

In the majority of kidneys the scarring due to chronic pyelonephritis and nephrosclerosis made the macroscopic diagnosis of amyloidosis unreliable, although firm waxy portions of surviving renal tissue were sometimes suggestive of this disease.

The kidney weights reflect this pattern. Only 41 combined weights were available. (The frequent preservation of the entire urinary tract for further study and photography explains this absence of reliable kidney weights.)

Under 10 oz	14 cases	Less than normal
10–15 oz	7 cases	Within normal limits
Over 15 oz	20 cases	Greater than normal

Other macroscopic findings in the kidneys from the 65 cases of amyloidosis included 27 cases of pyonephrosis, 11 cases of hydronephrosis and 12 cases with renal calculi.

Renal Vein Thrombosis. In his textbook on *Renal and Urinary Affections*, Dickinson in 1877 and 1885 described renal vein thrombosis in association with chronic disease of the kidney. He attributed the thrombosis to 'the hindrance which occurs to the circulation from the encroachment of fibroids,

growth, the pressure of distended tubules or the lardaceous thickening of the arterial coats'.

Harrison *et al.* (1956) described 11 cases of renal vein thrombosis secondary to renal disease and included 4 cases in which the thrombosis was associated with renal amyloidosis. Barclay *et al.* (1960) presented 9 new cases of renal vein thrombosis

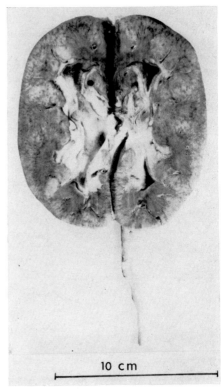

FIG. 6.4. Opened kidney to show the appearances of 'pure renal amyloidosis'. The kidney was twice normal size and weighed 300 g.

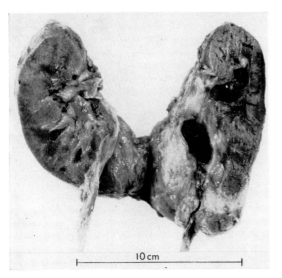

FIG. 6.5. Horseshoe kidney involved by 'pure renal amyloidosis'. The renal tissue has the characteristic pale, firm white waxy appearance suggestive of amyloidosis, and the left pelvis is dilated and inflamed from a terminal pyonephrosis. *See* Case History p. 102.

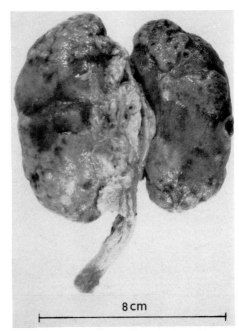

FIG. 6.7. External appearance of the kidney depicted in Fig. 6.6. There is only moderate scarring in the mid-zones corresponding to areas of chronic pyelonephritis.

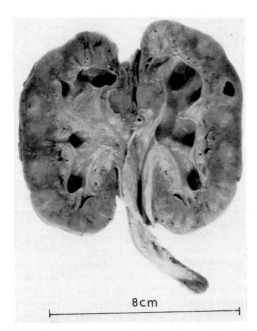

FIG. 6.6. Cut surface of a kidney from a thirty-six year old paraplegic who died in renal failure from severe renal amyloidosis and mild chronic pyelo-nephritis. Note the early hydronephrosis, lack of severe scarring, cortico-medullary blurring, and only slight reduction in renal tissue.

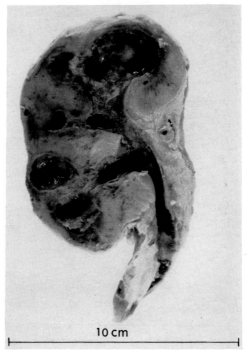

FIG. 6.8. Cut surface of a kidney showing a chronic pyonephrosis. This occurred as a late event in a thirty-nine year old paraplegic who died in renal failure from severe renal amyloidosis.

(5 bilateral and 4 unilateral), in association with (secondary) amyloid disease of the kidney, and were only able to find 39 previously recorded cases in the literature. They considered renal vein thrombosis an important, and often terminal, complication of amyloidosis of the kidneys and quoted Vilk (1940) who found 13 cases in 249 post-mortems of amyloid disease (approx. 1:20).

In the 65 cases of amyloidosis in this series, there were 3 of renal vein thrombosis (2 bilateral and 1 unilateral). This incidence agrees with the findings of Vilk, and suggests that although renal vein

MICROSCOPIC

Staining Methods

In all 65 cases there was no difficulty in staining the amyloid tissue by routine histological methods. There were no variations in staining as is found in some cases of primary amyloidosis.

The two most commonly used methods were—

1. The Congo Red method.
2. The methyl violet metachromatic method.

Considerable experience with these methods shows that, in spite of certain technical difficulties

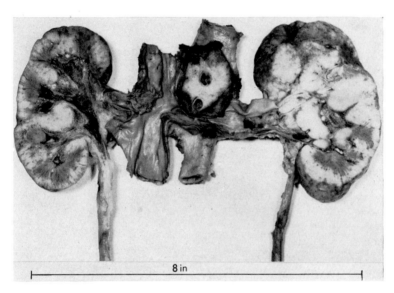

8 in

FIG. 6.9. Bilateral renal vein thrombosis associated with severe renal amyloidosis. Note the typical appearance of renal amyloid with scarring from mild chronic pyelonephritis. Both renal veins and their main tributaries are filled with thrombi, and on the right side the thrombus has extended into the inferior vena cava.

thrombosis may occur with renal amyloidosis it is an uncommon terminal event. Barclay and his co-workers suggested that the primary origin of the thrombi was at the capillary level as of their 9 cases, 7 had thrombi both in the small arcuate veins and within some glomerular capillaries. In contrast, the site of the thrombosis in our 3 cases was confined to the renal veins and their major tributories (*see* Fig. 6.9). With so few cases it is impossible to make any definite conclusion concerning this interesting and fatal complication of renal amyloidosis. Brief clinical and pathological details of our cases are shown in Table 6.9.

Adrenals

In severe involvement of the adrenals by amyloid material, these glands were enlarged from diffuse cortical thickening. Usually, it was impossible to diagnose adrenal amyloidosis at necropsy.

and the necessity of using a sugar mounting medium, the methyl violet method is superior. This superiority is especially valid when looking for small amounts of amyloid. With a properly stained methyl violet section there has been no doubt in the writer's experience as to the presence or absence of amyloid material. This is in contrast to the Congo Red method, where it is impossible to be certain about the presence of small amounts of amyloid due to the orange staining of other tissues. After trying several techniques the methyl violet method of Fernando (1961) was found to be superior, and was used for the detection of amyloid throughout the series.

Two new, but not necessarily better, methods have been recently introduced. First, Vassar and Culling (1959, 1962) found that both primary and secondary amyloid fluoresced specifically when stained with Thioflavine T. Kurban (1960) found this method useful to the skin histopathologist, and Hobbs and

TABLE 6.9

Renal vein thrombosis and amyloidosis in chronic paraplegia

(Incidence: 3 cases (2 bilateral and 1 unilateral) in 65 cases of amyloidosis)

Case no	Sex	Age at death	Cause of paraplegia	Level of paraplegia	Survival time since paraplegia	Pressure sores	Osteo-myelitis	Terminal Blood Urea	Clinical features	Degree of amyloid in kidney	Cause of death
128	Male	55	Trauma—road traffic accident	Cauda-equina incomplete	6 years	+ + +	—	320	Admitted to hospital 2 days before death in acute renal failure	+ + +	I. Renal failure due to bilateral renal vein thrombosis, and amyloidosis*
166	Male	53	Trauma—mining accident	L1/2 complete	24½ years	+ + +	+ + +	110	Heart failure from repeated myocardial infarcts. Diabetes mellitus for 11 years. No suspicion of amyloidosis	+ +	I. Old and recent myocardial infarction due to severe coronary heart disease. II. Bilateral renal vein thrombosis due to amyloidosis
196	Male	43	'Arach-noiditis'	T5 complete	13 years	+ + +	+ + +	368	Rapid development of severe nephrosis and uraemia. Mild hypertension for one year	+ + +	I. Renal failure due to amyloidosis, and unilateral renal vein thrombosis II. Mild hypertensive heart disease

* Upper urinary tract illustrated in Fig. 6.9.

Morgan (1963) thought it preferable to other methods. McKinney and Grubb (1965) found a high incidence of false positives with this stain. In our experience certain difficulties were found in detecting amyloid in the rectum (Arapakis and Tribe, 1963), but in all other tissues it produced as clear and distinctive a picture as the methyl violet stain. Second, Heller *et al.* (1964) detected amyloid in Congo Red stained sections with the polarising microscope and claimed that it reveals small deposits of amyloid material undetectable by ordinary methods. We have not been able to confirm these findings.

Methods Used for the Histological Grading of Amyloid

With the possible exception of the kidneys, all organs involved in secondary amyloidosis show an even distribution of this material throughout their structure. For this reason, the amount of amyloid seen in one histological section from any organ is representative of the amount to be found throughout that organ. On this basis, two methods of histological grading were employed.

First, each organ was graded quantitatively from 0 to + + + on the amount of amyloid seen on microscopy. Second, each case was graded from I to III on the basis of the amount of amyloid detected throughout the body.

Details of the grading methods are given in Tables 6.10 and 6.11.

TABLE 6.10

Method A (Histological grading of Individual organs)

Grade 0	Tissue stained for amyloid but none detected
Grade ±	Definite, but very slight amyloid present
Grade +	Definite amyloid present, usually confined to vessel walls
Grade + +	Moderately severe involvement with amyloid
Grade + + +	Almost complete replacement of the organ examined by amyloid

NB + + + recorded in kidneys implies complete replacement of the glomerular tufts by amyloid.

The results of Grading Method *A* will be given in the next section of this chapter when describing the changes produced by amyloidosis in individual organs.

TABLE 6.11

Method B (Histological grading of individual cases)

Grade I	Anything up to and including one organ with + +
Grade II	At least two organs with + + and not more than one with + + +
Grade III	At least two organs with + + +

On the basis of Grading Method *B* the 65 cases were grouped as follows—

Grade   I   11 cases
Grade II   40 cases
Grade III   14 cases

The significance of the results of this grading method will be examined in the section devoted to discussing the distribution of amyloid in this series (p. 85).

The findings in individual organs are now described in detail. In most articles on amyloidosis the pathological findings are restricted to four organs—the kidneys, liver, spleen, and the adrenal glands and the changes in these organs will be described first. Table 6.12 summarises the findings.

TABLE 6.12

Microscopic distribution of amyloid in the kidneys, spleen, liver, and adrenals

Tissue	0	± and +	++	+++	Sections available
Kidney	0	14	12	37	63
Spleen	1	15	34	12	62
Liver	0	29	29	4	62
Adrenals	0	19	24	4	47

KIDNEYS

The histological patterns of amyloid deposition in the kidneys in this series agreed basically with the classical descriptions of Auerbach and Stemmerman (1944a, 1944b). They divided their cases into minimal, moderate, and advanced renal amyloidosis primarily on glomerular involvement. In addition, they described amyloid deposition around the tubules (peritubular amyloid) and within the walls of the renal vessels (vascular amyloid). The distribution in these three sites in the 63 cases with adequate histological material in this series is shown in Table 6.13.

TABLE 6.13

Sites of amyloid deposition in the kidneys (63 cases)

Site	0	± and +	++	+++
Glomerular	0	14	12	37
Peritubular	4	21	38	*
Vascular	6	28	29	†

* The peritubular amyloid was usually deposited around the medullary tubules; it never completely replaced these structures.

† The vascular amyloid was seen chiefly in the walls of the small and medium sized cortical vessels. There was never complete replacement of the walls of the larger arteries.

Photomicrographs of the typical features of renal amyloidosis are shown in Figs. 6.10 and 6.11, and no further description of these classical findings is required.

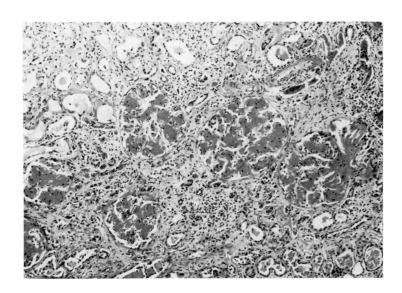

Fig. 6.10. Severe glomerular involvement in typical renal amyloidosis. The tubular changes are secondary to the glomerular amyloidosis and there is no pyelonephritis. H & E. ×120.

However, the classical picture of renal amyloidosis in this series was complicated by the frequent coexistence of chronic pyelonephritis. In the 63 cases with kidney tissue available for microscopy, the following degrees of chronic pyelonephritis were found—

Nil	5 cases	Slight	28 cases
Moderate	16 cases	Severe	14 cases

In only 5 was there no evidence of pyelonephritis, and in these the histological pattern agreed completely with the classical description of 'pure' renal amyloidosis. In a further 28, there was only slight chronic pyelonephritis and in these, when the amyloid involvement was severe, it was undoubtedly the chief factor causing renal failure.

In the remaining 30 cases, the chronic pyelonephritis was either moderate or severe, and the classical microscopic picture of these two conditions was chiefly altered by unique glomerular changes. If the chronic pyelonephritis had reached the atrophic stage with complete hyalinisation of the glomeruli, then amyloid material was not deposited in these structures. If, however, there were any surviving capillaries in the glomerular tufts, then the amyloid was deposited around these vessels and eventually obliterated them (*see* Figs. 5.10 and 5.14). The peritubular and vascular amyloid patterns were only distorted by the amount of remaining interstitial tissue, i.e. no amyloid was deposited around the 'thyroid' tubules of atrophic chronic pyelonephritis. Vascular amyloid deposition often obscured the nephrosclerotic changes and, in particular, it was impossible to distinguish the fibrinoid necrosis of malignant nephrosclerosis if amyloid was present (Fig. 6.12).

The kidneys involved by both chronic pyelonephritis and amyloidosis could be divided into two fairly clear cut types—

1. Kidneys chiefly involved by amyloidosis in which there was frequently evidence of acute pyelonephritis occurring as a terminal event.
2. Kidneys chiefly involved by atrophic chronic pyelonephritis in which amyloid deposition in the surviving glomeruli appeared to be the terminal event, leading directly to complete renal failure.

The combination of amyloidosis and active chronic pyelonephritis was not common.

All previous writers have stated that the first histological evidence of renal amyloidosis is involvement of the glomerular capillaries. However, in this series, in addition to amyloid situated in the classical sites, several kidneys have shown 'cortical masses' of amyloid material unrelated to any renal structures. These were usually situated beneath the capsule and were often lying within areas of active chronic pyelonephritis. Although commonly associated with amyloid deposition in the classical sites, in at least 4 kidneys (2 from post-mortem cases and 2 removed from paraplegics during life), these masses were the only evidence of amyloidosis in the kidneys. Situated usually in the renal tissue directly beneath the kidney capsule, these 'cortical masses' appeared to be localised deposits of amyloid produced in direct response to renal suppuration. The masses were usually about three to five times the size of a

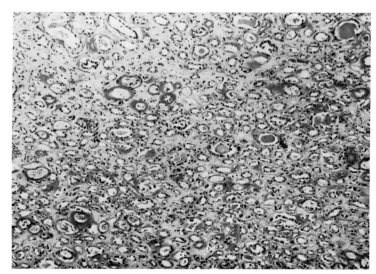

FIG. 6.11. Peritubular involvement in typical renal amyloidosis. There is focal deposition of amyloid material around the tubules with a generalized interstitial fibrosis. H & E. ×120.

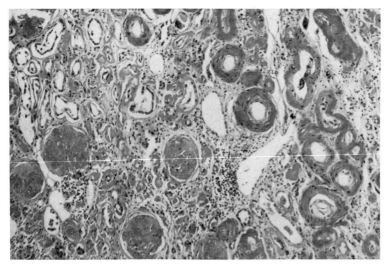

FIG. 6.12. Chronic pyelonephritis, hypertension, and renal amyloidosis. The glomeruli are partially sclerosed from chronic pyelonephritis with complete amyloid replacement of the surviving glomerular tufts. The renal vessels show endarteritis fibrosa, but the severe amyloid infiltration of their walls obscures any evidence of fibrinoid necrosis. H & E. ×108.

glomerulus and, although usually subcortical, they also occurred in the deeper parts of the cortex and the medulla, in relation to areas of active chronic pyelonephritis (Fig. 6.13). In one nephrectomy specimen the appearances were particularly striking. This kidney showed almost confluent active chronic pyelonephritis and xanthogranulomatous foreign-body reaction around the pelvis and calyces (Fig. 6.14). Microscopy showed slight amyloid infiltration of occasional glomerular capillaries and small cortical arteries, and a layer of subcapsular 'cortical masses' of amyloid so numerous that they were easily visible on naked-eye inspection of a methyl violet stained slide (Figs. 6.15 and 6.16).

One post-mortem case is worth special mention as it provided further evidence to support this theory of local amyloid deposition in response to renal suppuration.

Case History

T. M. (Case no. 186) aged fifty-six at the time of his death, suffered a traumatic paraplegia one and a half years previously with a resulting incomplete lesion at C.4–C.6. He was admitted to Stoke Mandeville Hospital the day after injury, and made normal progress on routine treatment. He was finally transferred to another hospital after ten and a half months, never having had pressure sores and with only a mild urinary infection. He was re-admitted four days before his death with gross deep pressure sores over the sacrum and both trochanters eroding the underlying bones. He was extremely ill, and died with a terminal blood urea of 170 mg per cent.

At post-mortem, the heart was slightly enlarged and there were small friable endocardial vegetations on all four heart valves with no evidence of previous cardiac disease. The lungs showed acute pulmonary oedema and cultures of the blood, vegetations, and lung tissue all grew a haemolytic streptococcus (Group C). The kidneys were acutely swollen with some shallow scars at both poles of the left kidney. On microscopy, there were generalised non-specific changes in the kidneys compatible with septicaemia and special stains revealed mild amyloid deposition in the glomerular tufts on both sides. However, the scarred areas of the left kidney showed active chronic pyelonephritis with numerous large 'cortical masses' of amyloid material. Small amounts of amyloid were also demonstrated in the thyroid, heart, liver, spleen, adrenals, prostate, and bladder. Some mesenteric lymph nodes and the intestinal tract showed moderate amyloid deposition. No amyloid could be demonstrated in sections from the pressure sores.

Comment

This case shows several interesting points—

1. Septicaemia and acute streptococcal endocarditis of all four heart valves, presumably arising from gross pressure sores.
2. The development of early generalised amyloidosis within seven and a half months of developing pressure sores.
3. Localised 'cortical masses' of amyloid that were confined to the focal regions of one kidney involved by active chronic pyelonephritis.

Further analysis of the post-mortem series revealed a further 20 cases in which the kidneys showed varying numbers of cortical amyloid masses with different degrees of normally distributed amyloid. Of these, 15 had evidence of severe chronic pyelonephritis, 3 showed slight pyelonephritis, and in only 2 was there no evidence of pyelonephritis in the

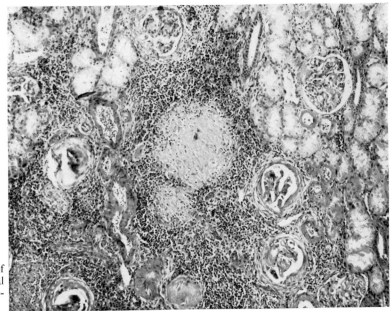

FIG. 6.13. Local deposition of amyloid masses within a focal area of active chronic pyelonephritis. H & E. ×108.

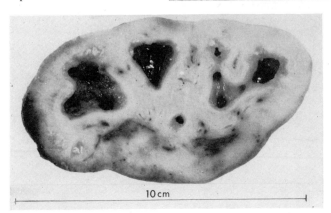

10 cm

FIG. 6.14. Cut surface of a (non-functioning) kidney, removed during life from a female paraplegic, showing a chronic pyonephrosis. The small yellow, almost confluent, abscesses visible in the tissues around the calyces showed the changes of xanthogranulomatous pyelonephritis depicted in Figs. 5.11 and 5.12. In addition, microscopy of this kidney showed widespread active chronic pyelonephritis with numerous 'cortical masses' of amyloid.

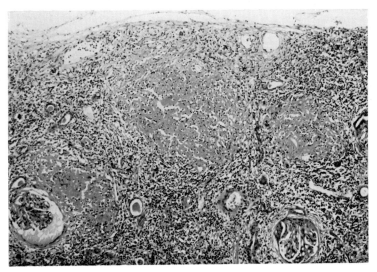

FIG. 6.15. Section from beneath the capsule of the kidney illustrated in Fig. 6.14 showing several large 'cortical masses' of amyloid associated with active chronic pyelonephritis. H & E. ×120.

sections available. These figures suggest that renal suppuration can lead to the deposition of localised masses of amyloid before contributing, with other aetiological factors, to the generalised deposition of amyloid throughout the body. No evidence has been found elsewhere in this series of amyloid being

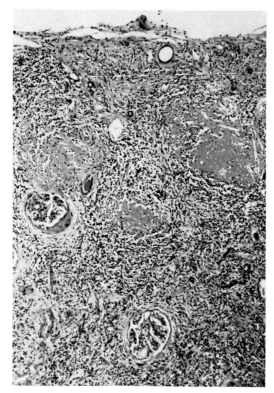

FIG. 6.16. A further section from the kidney illustrated in Fig. 6.14. This shows how the local 'cortical masses' of amyloid were restricted in this kidney to the sub-capsular region. There is also almost complete tubular destruction from active chronic pyelone-phritis. H & E. ×120.

deposited in response to chronic infection, i.e. there has been no evidence of amyloid in many surgical specimens of excised chronic pressure sores and sinuses.

The aetiology of renal amyloidosis in this series can be summarised in Fig. 6.17.

Although the processes 1, 2 and 3 in Fig. 6.17 could occasionally be recognised as acting individually in the cause of renal amyloidosis in this series, a combination of two or all three processes was commonly found.

In this series amyloidosis was thought only to cause death by involvement of the kidneys. For this

reason a more detailed description has been given of amyloid deposition in the kidneys than in other organs. Within the kidneys, it is involvement of the glomeruli that leads directly to renal failure and, consequently, grading of renal amyloid was made solely on the degree of replacement of the glomerular tufts by myloid material. When in any one case all the surviving glomeruli were completely replaced by amyloid, irrespective of the degree of chronic pyelonephritis, this case was graded +++ and the amyloid was considered to have played the major part in the resulting renal failure. On this basis, the part played by amyloidosis in the causes of death of the 63 patients, with available kidney tissue for histology, was assessed in Table 6.14. The very high

TABLE 6.14

The part played by amyloidosis in renal failure in chronic paraplegia

Amyloidosis the major cause of death	37 patients (59%)
Amyloidosis a contributory cause of death	16 patients
Amyloidosis present, but played no part in the cause of death	10 patients

proportion of severe involvement of the kidneys in comparison with other organs was a striking feature of this series and will be discussed later.

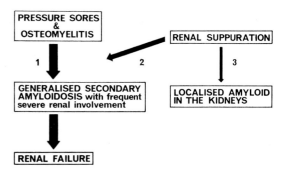

FIG. 6.17. Aetiology of renal amyloidosis in chronic paraplegia.

SPLEEN

The degree of amyloid infiltration in the spleen in this series is shown in Table 6.12. The histological picture showed no basic differences from the classical descriptions. There appeared to be equal numbers of 'focal' and 'diffuse' types of amyloid deposition, with a few cases showing only slight involvement of the small vessels.

LIVER

In comparison with the kidneys, a feature in this series was the infrequent severe involvement of the liver (*see* Table 6.12). In only 4 cases was the liver almost completely replaced by amyloid tissue (Grade + + +), and 2 of these were unassociated with the septic complications of paraplegia (i.e. these were the cases associated with tuberculosis and neuroblastoma). On microscopy, the amyloid deposition in the liver usually fell into two distinct patterns. Using the precedent set by Levine (1962), these have been termed parenchymal and vascular.

In the parenchymal form the first sign of amyloid was deposition around the sinusoidal capillaries between the liver cells. As this type progressed in severity, the amyloid tissue increased with compression and atrophy of the liver cells. Often there was almost complete destruction of the liver cells before any amyloid was deposited in the walls of the periportal vessels (Fig. 6.18).

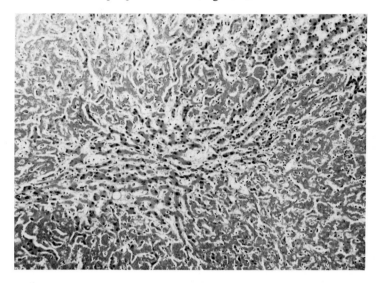

FIG. 6.18. Severe amyloid deposition in the liver of the parenchymal type. The amyloid has destroyed at least two-thirds of the liver parenchymal cells, but the vessels are not involved. H & E. ×120.

In the more common vascular form, the earliest stage was deposition of amyloid within the walls of the periportal vessels, and the great majority of cases grade ± or + were of this type and showed no amyloid deposition within the sinusoids (Fig. 6.19).

In only a few cases (grade + +), was there a mixed parenchymal and vascular type of amyloid deposition. In these the amyloid deposited in the parenchymal

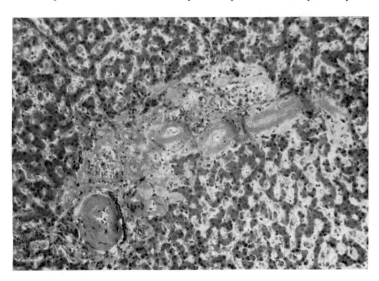

FIG. 6.19. Amyloid deposition in the liver of the vascular type. The amyloid material is restricted to the walls of the portal vessels, and there is no alteration of the liver parenchymal cells. H & E. ×150.

and vascular sites usually showed a slight but distinct difference in metachromatic staining, suggesting that the amyloid in these different sites may have a different biochemical structure.

Jaundice is a very rare accompaniment of hepatic amyloidosis (Orloff and Felder, 1946), and in no case in this series did amyloidosis appear to upset hepatic function. In contrast, Dietrick and Russi (1958) attributed death to hepatic involvement in 2 of 6 patients with paraplegia who died from amyloidosis.

ADRENALS

The amyloid deposition in the adrenals showed a similar pattern of severity to that found in the liver and spleen (Table 6.12). There were only 4 cases of almost complete replacement, all occurring in cases with septic complications of paraplegia. As in the liver and spleen, the histological picture was basically

Guttman (1930) studied 566 cases of Addison's disease and attributed 7 to amyloidosis. However, Stemmerman and Auerbach (1944) in a study of 468 cases of generalised amyloidosis found involvement of the adrenals in 354 (81%), severe in 94 (21%), but were unable to find indubitable clinical signs of Addison's disease in any case. They suggested certain subclinical signs of adrenal hypofunction but gave no biochemical proof. None of the cases in this series showed clinical evidence of Addison's disease. However, in view of the fairly frequent moderate and severe involvement of the adrenal glands by amyloid, a detailed biochemical study is indicated in further cases for adrenal hypofunction has been suggested as a possible cause of testicular atrophy in paraplegics. It will be shown later that all the endocrine glands can be involved by secondary amyloidosis and, with the advent of more sophis-

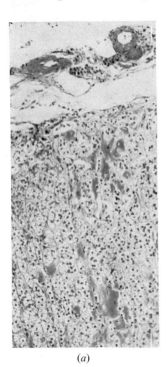 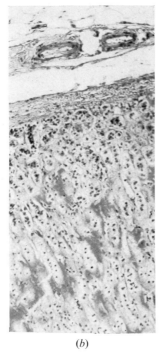

(a) (b)

FIG. 6.20. Adrenal amyloidosis.

(a) Vascular pattern: the amyloid is deposited in the walls of the periadrenal vessels and also between the cortical cells.

(b) Parenchymal pattern: the amyloid is restricted to the adrenal cortex with no vascular involvement. H & E. ×108.

similar to the classical descriptions. However, a distinction could be made between parenchymal and vascular types of amyloid deposition. This was not quite so clear as in the liver, and was based chiefly on the presence or absence of amyloid infiltration of the periadrenal vessels. The distinction was usually obvious, but the periadrenal vessels were rarely involved alone; usually there was involvement of the adrenal cortex at the same time (Figs. 6.20a and b).

ticated tests of endocrine function, serial investigation of these cases would be of great value and interest.

The four organs so far described, kidneys, liver, spleen, and adrenals, are usually the only organs described in articles on amyloidosis. However, it is well recognised that, if looked for, amyloid can be detected in many other organs. It was thought worthwhile to look for amyloid in all the histological material available in these cases. The results are shown in Table 6.15.

TABLE 6.15

Microscopic distribution of amyloid in other tissues of the body

Tissue	0	Grade ± and +	++	Sections available
Heart	6	42	1	49
Thyroid	3	25	13	41
Pancreas	1	35	4	40
Lungs	27	7	0	34
Brain	15	0	0	15
Pituitary	3	12	4	19
Gastro-intestinal tract	0	15	18	33
Testis	15	10	2	27
Prostate	7	10	1	18
Bladder	10	5	0	15
Lymph nodes	4	6	2	12
Choroid plexus	0	8	1	9
Salivary glands	0	4	4	8
Bone marrow	3	2	0	5
Parathyroid	0	3	1	4

Amyloid was also detected in the aorta (3 cases), gall bladder (2 cases), ureter (2 cases), and seminal vesicles (1 case).

HEART

Involvement of the heart in primary amyloidosis is well recognised (Symmers, 1956), and amyloid cardiomyopathy is not infrequently described in these cases. Since in several patients in this series cardiac abnormalities during life had been attributed to amyloid involvement of the heart, particular attention was paid to this organ. Sections from the heart in 49 cases were stained for amyloid, and mild involvement was detected in 42 cases. In one case, there was moderate involvement. The amyloid was usually found in the walls of the small blood vessels within the myocardium, and there were frequently small deposits in the connective tissue beneath the endocardium. In several cases, focal areas could be found in which there was a delicate lace-like deposition around the individual muscle fibres (Fig. 6.21) similar to that described by Pomerance (1966) in senile cardiac amyloidosis. There were no cases with great masses of amyloid in the myocardium as is sometimes found in primary amyloidosis, and it is most unlikely that any of these sedentary patients suffered from any functional disability of their heart due to amyloidosis.

THYROID

Walker (1942) reviewed the literature on amyloid goitre and found 56 cases, but no evidence of reported thyroid insufficiency. In this series amyloid was detected in 38 of 41 sections of thyroid available. In 13, the amyloid deposition was moderately severe and appeared to have caused compression of

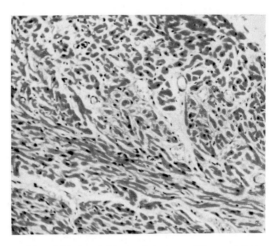

FIG. 6.21. Amyloidosis of the heart. The amyloid is focally deposited as a delicate lacework around the muscle fibres. H & E. ×108.

the thyroid acini. In all cases, the amyloid appeared first as a fine rim apparently laid down on the outer aspect of the follicular basement membrane. Gradually, this increased in thickness and eventually there appeared to be considerable compression and atrophy of the thyroid follicles (Fig. 6.22). No cases of clinical hypothyroidism were seen.

PANCREAS

Amyloid was detected in 39 of 40 sections of pancreas available. In the majority of these it was seen only in the walls of the smaller pancreatic blood vessels. In 4, however, there was infiltration beneath the epithelium of the pancreatic ducts with focal areas of periacinar involvement. Occasionally, amyloid was seen in the small vessels within Islets of Langerhans, but there never appeared to be compression of these structures.

LUNGS

Surprisingly, the lungs appeared to be resistant to amyloid deposition and small amounts in the pulmonary vessels were detected in only 7 of 34 cases. This is in contrast to generalised primary amyloidosis

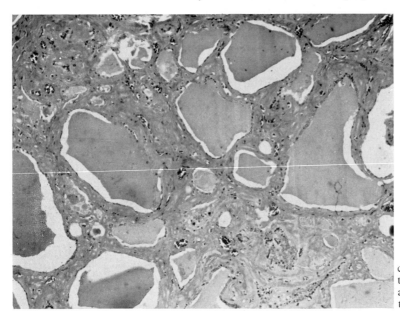

FIG. 6.22. Moderate perifollicular amyloid infiltration of the thyroid gland with compression and destruction of glandular tissue. H & E. ×108.

(Symmers, 1956), and also to generalised secondary amyloidosis associated with rheumatoid arthritis (Tribe, 1966) in which moderate deposition appears to be fairly common.

BRAIN AND CHOROID PLEXUS

Symmers (1956) noted that the central nervous system is invariably free from involvement in generalised amyloidosis, apart from the meningeal and choroid plexus vessels. The findings in this series

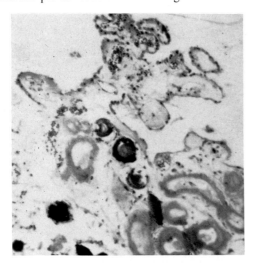

FIG. 6.23. Amyloid infiltration in the vessels of the choroid plexus. Some calcification is also present. H & E. ×150.

confirm this statement. No amyloid was found in sections from the brains of 15 cases, but in all 9 choroid plexuses examined amyloid could be detected in the walls of the small vessels (Fig. 6.23).

PITUITARY

In contrast, amyloid was detected in 16 of the 19 pituitary glands available for study. In the anterior lobes amyloid was laid down between the cells, and in 4 cases this appeared to have caused definite compression and atrophy of this part of the gland (Fig. 6.24a). In the posterior lobes the amyloid was restricted to the walls of the small vessels, and this also occurred in the vessels of the pituitary stalk (Fig. 6.24b).

GASTRO-INTESTINAL TRACT

In view of the current interest in rectal biopsy as a means of diagnosing amyloidosis, it is important to note that portions of the gastro-intestinal tract were stained for amyloid in 33 cases. Although amyloid was not detectable at all levels in every case, amyloid was present at some level in every case. An analysis of the different sites is shown in Table 6.16.

Apart from the literature on rectal biopsy, no references have been found giving any detailed pathological description of secondary amyloidosis of the gastro-intestinal tract. The author (Tribe, 1966) described the changes found in the gastro-intestinal tract in amyloidosis in rheumatoid arthritis, and compared them with the changes in amyloidosis associated with the septic complications

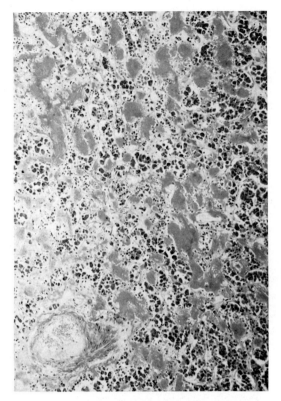 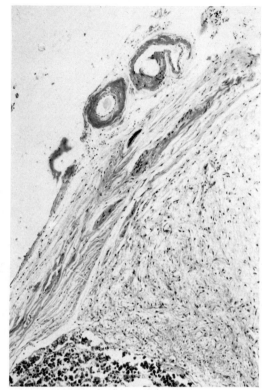

(*a*) Anterior lobe: large masses of amyloid can be seen lying between the anterior pituitary cells with compression, and destruction of nearly half the glandular tissue. H & E. × 120.

(*b*) Posterior lobe: amyloid deposition is restricted to the walls of vessels in the capsule and the pituitary stalk. H & E. × 120.

FIG. 6.24. Amyloidosis of the pituitary gland.

TABLE 6.16

Amyloidosis of the gastro-intestinal tract in chronic paraplegia
(Analysis of material from 33 cases)

Grade of amyloid	Site						
	Tongue	Oesophagus	Stomach	Duodenum	Small intestine	Large intestine	Rectum
0	1	3	1	0	3	4	2
± and +	15	7	11	10	7	10	8
++ and +++	0	0	12	5	14	8	1
Totals	16	10	24	15	24	22	11

of paraplegia. At that time it was noted that the difference between parenchymal and vascular involvement was often striking. With the exception of the tongue, where amyloid was always deposited around the mucous glands (Fig. 6.25) and sometimes as a thin rim beneath the surface epithelium, this distinction was usually clear cut.

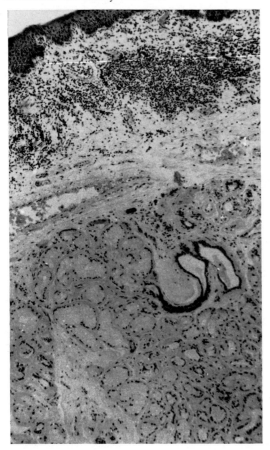

FIG. 6.25. Amyloidosis of the tongue. There is extensive amyloid deposition around the mucous glands of the tongue. H & E. ×108.

With pure vascular involvement, amyloid material was always found in the walls of the small vessels in the sub-mucosa throughout the gastro-intestinal tract and could, occasionally, be detected in the small vessels at the base of the mucosa and in the vessels in the muscle and serosal coats.

With pure parenchymal involvement the pattern of amyloid deposition was sufficiently definite to be termed 'classical' (Tribe, 1966). Figure 6.26 shows the topographical change in amyloid deposition throughout the length of the gut. In the stomach, the amyloid is distributed throughout the whole depth of the lamina propria (stroma) of the mucosa; in the small intestine only the inner half (i.e. closer to the lumen) is involved; in the large intestine the inner fifth; and in the rectum only a thin rim of amyloid material lies beneath the superficial (luminal) epithelium. Apart from Targgart *et al.* (1963), who noticed this progressive diminution of amyloid tissue along the whole length of the intestine in a case of systemic amyloidosis and ulcerative colitis, no other authors appear to have described this histological picture. Most authors have found amyloid within the walls of the submucosal vessels, and there are occasional references to smaller amounts in the lamina propria and between the muscle coats. Tribe (1966) suggested a dietary factor, absorbed in decreasing amounts as it travels down the gut, as a possible explanation of the 'classical' parenchymal pattern.

There were a few cases of mixed vascular and parenchymal deposition, and occasional cases with diffuse infiltration between the fibres of the muscle coats. In the oesophagus, vascular involvement was clear cut, but parenchymal involvement was only represented by a thin rim of amyloid beneath the squamous epithelium. In the duodenum, while the parenchymal deposition was usually similar to that in the small intestine, there was always deposition around Brunner's glands. In nearly all cases, the pattern of deposition (vascular or parenchymal) followed that in other organs of the body. In 20 cases amyloid was detected at sufficient levels throughout the gut to assess the pattern of distribution, and the results are compared with those in 5 cases of amyloidosis in rheumatoid arthritis in Table 6.17. In the remaining 13 cases, with only scanty material at one or two levels, the findings suggested the following patterns: Parenchymal—5 cases, parenchymal and vascular—6 cases, and vascular—2 cases.

TABLE 6.17

Site of amyloid deposition in secondary amyloidosis of the gastro-intestinal tract

	Paraplegic group (20 cases)	Arthritis group (5 cases)
Purely vascular	2	3
Vascular and parenchymal	3	1
Purely parenchymal	15	1

Using this material, Tribe (1966) considered that biopsy of the rectum should have a 90 per cent accuracy rate and suggested that biopsy of the stomach might have an even higher accuracy and should detect the few cases missed by rectal biopsy. It is also significant that in all cases in which amyloid was detected in the large intestine or rectum the major viscera, including the kidneys, were involved. Therefore, if amyloid is detected in the rectum it is almost certain that the kidneys are already involved.

investigation of renal function. The technique was to deprive the patient of fluids and food from 1900 hours; at 0800 the next morning a sample of blood was taken. The osmolarity was estimated on an advanced osmometer. The patient then drank a litre of water, further samples of blood were taken at half-hourly intervals, and their osmolarity determined. The results are expressed graphically (Fig. 6.27) with the results of a control patient. There is a rapid fall in the osmolarity of the blood by up to

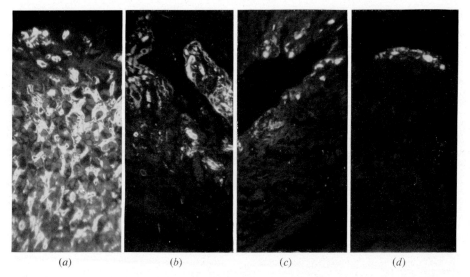

    (a)   (b)   (c)   (d)

FIG. 6.26. Amyloidosis of the gastro-intestinal tract. (*a*) Stomach, (*b*) small intestine, (*c*) colon, (*d*) rectum. Photomicrographs from different levels of the gastro-intestinal tract showing 'classical' parenchymal deposition of amyloid as described in the text. Thioflavine T fluorescent stain × 150. (Reproduced by permission from *Modern Trends in Rheumatology*, 1966, edited by Alan G. S. Hill. London: Butterworths.)

This is important since Arapakis and Tribe (1963) detected amyloid in the rectum of 3 cases of rheumatoid arthritis without proteinuria, and the latter can no longer be considered a reliable 'first sign' of amyloidosis. Unfortunately, there appears to be no correlation between the sites of amyloid involvement in the gastro-intestinal tract and the rate or extent of renal involvement.

It has been suggested (Symmers, 1956; Pidgeon, 1958; Comarr, 1963) that amyloidosis of the gut may be a cause of diarrhoea, malabsorption, and malnutrition. This was not observed in this series, apart from terminally when the patients died of uraemia. Absorption studies of water were carried out by Dr Silver in 5 patients with amyloidosis. The absorption studies were carried out as part of an

ten points in all the patients. This remained depressed for some hours. The fall in the osmolarity indicated that the water had been absorbed rapidly across the gut, and thus diluted the serum constituents. Subsequently, as the water was redistributed throughout all the tissue compartments, there was a gradual return to normal. In this small group of patients, therefore, amyloidosis did not interfere with absorption of water from the gastro-intestinal tract.

TESTIS AND PROSTATE

Both these organs showed vascular amyloid involvement in about half the cases examined. In occasional cases, amyloid material was also laid down around

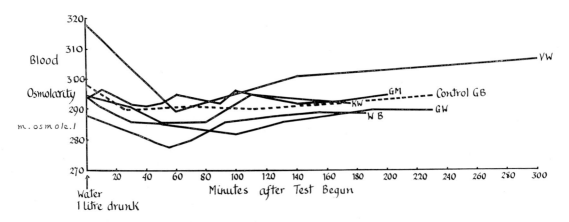

FIG. 6.27. Serial studies of the osmolarity of the blood in five paraplegics with generalised amyloidosis and one control patient. Results described in text.

the testicular tubules and the prostatic acini, but there never appeared to be any true compression of these structures (Fig. 6.28).

BLADDER

Of the 15 bladders examined only 5 showed mild involvement of the submucosal vessels. This is in marked contrast to amyloidosis in rheumatoid arthritis where the amyloid deposition is often widespread through the connective tissue of the submucosa and muscle coats and has been the cause of death through profuse haematuria in at least 2 known cases (Missen and Tribe, 1968).

LYMPH NODES

There have been no reports of the diagnosis of secondary amyloidosis by lymph node biopsy, but Mackenzie (1963) described the diagnosis of 3 cases of primary amyloidosis by this means. Only 12 lymph nodes, all from within the abdominal cavity, were examined in this series. Amyloid was detected in 8 and was severe in 2. Recollecting Teilums' theory (1964) that amyloid is a local secretion by pyronophilic reticulo-endothelial cells, more attention should be paid to amyloid deposition in lymphoid tissue. It would also be useful for diagnostic purposes to examine peripheral lymph nodes in cases of generalised amyloidosis.

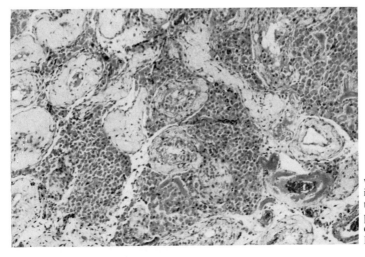

FIG. 6.28. Amyloid infiltration in the walls of small vessels in the testis. There is also complete atrophy of the testicular tubules and marked Leydig cell hyperplasia. These findings are common in chronic paraplegia (Tribe, 1963b). H & E. ×120.

SALIVARY GLANDS

Amyloid was detected in all eight salivary glands examined in this series, and in four the deposition was moderate to severe with considerable compression and atrophy of the glandular tissue (Fig. 6.29).

BONE-MARROW

Conn and Sundberg (1961) were able to detect amyloid material in bone marrow smears and sections from aspirated particles in cases of both primary and secondary amyloidosis. In the few cases examined in this series, it was restricted to the walls of small vessels and in no cases did it appear to be sufficient to interfere with haemopoiesis.

PARATHYROIDS

These endocrine glands can also be involved and amyloid was detected in all 4 cases examined. The deposition was parenchymal in type, between the glandular cells, and in one case was moderately severe with compression and some atrophy of the gland (Fig. 6.30).

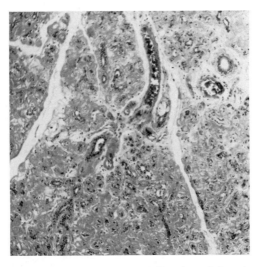

FIG. 6.29. Severe amyloid infiltration of the submandibular gland, with almost complete compression atrophy of the glandular acini. H & E. ×108.

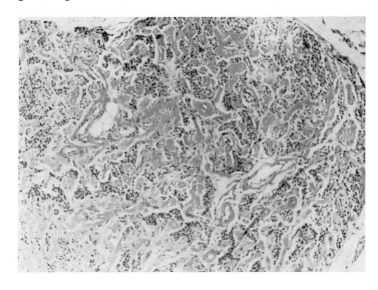

FIG. 6.30. Amyloid infiltration of the parathyroid gland with considerable compression atrophy. H & E. ×120.

Discussion on the Distribution of Amyloid in this Series

In studying these cases, certain peculiarities of amyloid distribution were noted both throughout the body and within individual organs.

Amyloid Distribution Throughout the Body

As shown in Table 6.12, the kidneys were more prone to severe involvement than other major viscera. If this is peculiar to amyloidosis associated with paraplegia, it obviously has a grave prognostic significance. Briggs (1961) also found a high incidence of severe renal amyloidosis in cases of amyloidosis in paraplegics. He found that 15 of 24 such cases had died from renal failure and commented that, although they all showed associated chronic pyelonephritis, the amyloidosis played a significant part in the renal failure in every case. More recently,

Dalton *et al.* (1965) reported 18 deaths directly due to renal failure out of 26 paraplegic patients with amyloidosis.

The literature, where specific, indicates a lower incidence of renal failure in other series. Auerbach and Stemmerman studied 468 necropsies performed on cases of amyloidosis, 463 of which were due to tuberculosis. They found evidence of amyloid in the kidneys in 379 (83%) and considered that 119 died in uraemia or pre-uraemia. They stated specifically 'that in the majority of cases the extent of the amyloid involvement of the kidneys lags behind that of the liver and spleen'. The cases usually die from tuberculosis and only in prolonged or healing cases does the amyloidosis lead to nephrosis and uraemia'. Cohen (1943), in a series of 79 patients with amyloidosis from tuberculosis, found only 5 patients (6%) who died in uraemia. In contrast, Powell and Swan (1955) found 19 out of 50 (38%) patients, with amyloidosis due to leprosy, died from renal failure. Dixon (1934), in a smaller series of more varied aetiology, considered that only 12 of 46 cases showed renal insufficiency.

Two cases in this series were not due to the septic complications of paraplegia. One was due to tuberculosis and the other was associated with widespread neuroblastoma. Both these cases had Grade III amyloidosis, yet both had only early renal involvement. Neither died from renal failure and the amyloid distribution throughout the organs of both cases was predominantly parenchymal. Brief case histories are of interest.

1. E. B. (Case no. 10) aged twenty-three at death, had a complete traumatic paraplegia at T.6 three years previously, and developed pulmonary tuberculosis and a tuberculous psoas abscess. At necropsy, death was due to his tuberculous infections with a terminal bronchopneumonia. In addition, there was generalised amyloidosis. Although he had developed some pressure sores following paraplegia he had no underlying osteomyelitis and there was no clinical or pathological evidence of severe pyelonephritis. His amyloidosis was therefore attributed to his tuberculosis. The amyloidosis involved both the liver and spleen (+++), but there was only early involvement of the kidneys (+). The amyloid deposition was parenchymal in type.

2. Miss D. W. (Case no. 147) aged twenty-one at death, developed a complete paraplegia in the mid-thoracic region two years previously. Laminectomy at that time revealed a 'small round-cell malignant tumour' surrounding the spinal cord thought to be compatible with lymphosarcoma. She was admitted to Stoke Mandeville Hospital eight months before her death. From this time the level of her paraplegia gradually rose up to C.5 and she developed bilateral malignant pleural effusions with increasing respiratory distress. She suffered only mild pressure sores and a mild cystitis. The diagnosis of amyloidosis was not considered during life.

At necropsy, the cause of death was due to pulmonary collapse due to pleural effusions and a huge mediastinal tumour mass. This had grown directly through the thoracic vertebrae to surround and compress the spinal cord. On microscopy it was considered to be a neuroblastoma, probably arising from the thoracic sympathetic nervous system. Surprisingly, she also had widespread secondary amyloidosis involving the following organs:

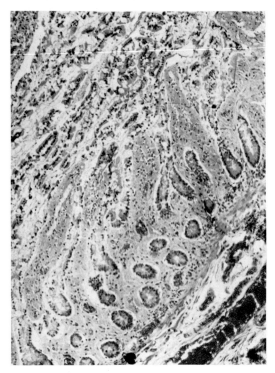

Fig. 6.31. Severe parenchymal amyloid infiltration in the mucosa of the small intestine. H & E. ×108. Miss D. W., Case no. 147. Case-history described in the text.

kidney +, liver +++, spleen +++, adrenal +, thyroid ±, pancreas ++, heart ++, small intestine +++ (Fig. 6.31), and large intestine ++. The kidneys showed only early involvement of the glomeruli, vessels and peritubular tissues and there was no evidence of pyelonephritis. In all these organs, parenchymal deposition predominated. The amyloidosis in this case, therefore, was considered to be of the rare secondary type associated with tumours. No previous reference to amyloidosis associated with neuroblastoma has been found.

The pattern of amyloid distribution in these 2 cases was so different from the cases associated with the septic complications of paraplegia that it was decided to study pathological material from cases of secondary amyloidosis not associated with paraplegia. Apart from these 2 cases, and 8 associated with chronic arthritis, no such material was available in this hospital. Therefore, with the kind permission of Dr Robb-Smith, histological material from 21 cases of secondary amyloidosis who died at the Radcliffe Infirmary, Oxford were studied. Of these, 13 were associated with tuberculosis and the remainder had a variety of secondary diseases (osteomyelitis 3, bronchiectasis 2, spinal abscesses 2, and carcinoma 1).

Table 6.18 shows a comparison between the patterns of amyloid distribution in 14 cases associated

preponderance of the parenchymal type of amyloid deposition in the organs.

Amyloid Distribution within Individual Organs

Two patterns of amyloid distribution within the individual organs could be distinguished in most cases in this series. Using the terminology of Levine (1962), these have been called parenchymal and vascular. Descriptions, where applicable, of these different sites of deposition in individual organs have been given earlier in this chapter. The distinction could most easily be made in the liver, adrenals, gastro-intestinal tract, and spleen. The pattern

TABLE 6.18
Amyloid distribution in cases of secondary amyloidosis associated with different diseases

Groups	No. of cases	Glomerular involvement with amyloid			Grade of amyloid throughout body			Site of amyloid distribution	
		+	++	+++	I	II	III	Parenchymal	Vascular
A. Amyloidosis associated with tuberculosis	14	7	3	4	1	9	4	13	1
B. Amyloidosis associated with paraplegia	61	12	11	38	10	39	12	26*	28*
C. Amyloidosis unassociated with either paraplegia or tuberculosis†	17	3	8	5	1	11	5	4	13

* Seven cases showed equal amounts of amyloid deposition in parenchymal and vascular sites.

† The underlying diseases in these cases were osteomyelitis (3), bronchiectasis (2), spinal abscesses (2), carcinoma (2), and chronic arthritis (8). The latter group have been studied before (Tribe, 1966) and showed that vascular deposition predominated in 7 of the 8 cases.

with tuberculosis, 61 cases associated with the septic complications of paraplegia, and 17 cases unassociated with either paraplegia or tuberculosis.

These cases were too few to enable any definite conclusion to be drawn. However, they do show that secondary amyloidosis is by no means a uniform disease and may run a different course according to the type of associated disease. It does seem certain that amyloidosis associated with the septic complications of paraplegia is accompanied by a higher incidence of severe renal involvement than amyloidosis associated with tuberculosis. Unfortunately the only large series of cases that have been available for study have been either secondary to paraplegia or to tuberculosis, so it has not been possible to confirm whether this picture is unique. In addition, the cases of amyloidosis associated with tuberculosis showed a

tended to be consistent throughout the organs in any one case and, although some amyloid was usually deposited in both sites, one or other pattern predominated. Of the 61 cases in this series in which there was sufficient histological material to differentiate these patterns, vascular deposition predominated in 28 cases, parenchymal in 26 and in 7 cases the amount of amyloid deposition appeared to be equal in the two sites. Thus, as distinct from amyloidosis due to tuberculosis in which the parenchymal pattern predominates, and amyloidosis associated with chronic arthritis in which the vascular pattern probably predominates (Tribe, 1966), there is no definite predominance of either pattern in paraplegics.

As noted before, a slight but definite difference in the metachromatic staining of the amyloid material deposited in the parenchymal and vascular sites on the liver has suggested a possible difference in chemical structure in these two sites, and this might be related to the different aetiological factors. However, there was no evidence to suggest that the vascular pattern was associated predominantly with kidney suppuration and the parenchymal with osteomyelitis, as, although 31 cases followed this distribution, an almost equal number, 28, did not. Nor was the vascular pattern more frequently found in cases with severe renal amyloidosis, and no relation could be found between the sites and rapidity of amyloid deposition.

At present, therefore, it is not understood why amyloid distribution in cases of secondary amyloidosis often shows such a clear cut distinction between parenchymal and vascular types. Although a clinical and morphological study such as this may never provide the complete answer to this problem, the distinction is of importance if only because a satisfactory theory of the pathogenesis of amyloidosis must explain the different morphological patterns.

To summarise the findings concerning amyloid distribution in this series—

1. Chronic pyelonephritis is sometimes associated with local deposition of amyloid forming 'cortical masses' not found in classical renal amyloidosis.

2. Irrespective of the degree of pyelonephritis, amyloidosis associated with paraplegia seems to produce more severe renal involvement with renal failure than secondary amyloidosis due to tuberculosis. Insufficient evidence, concerning amyloidosis associated with diseases other than tuberculosis or paraplegia, makes it impossible to be certain that this is unique to cases associated with paraplegia.

3. The distribution of amyloid within various organs in this series can be divided into parenchymal and vascular types. Although the latter type predominates compared with secondary amyloidosis from tuberculosis, there is no specific relationship to pyelonephritis, and this variation in pattern is at present not understood.

Hypertension and Amyloidosis

Of the 65 patients with amyloidosis, 31 had clinical and pathological evidence of hypertension, and the relationship of high blood pressure to chronic renal disease, including amyloidosis, in these patients will be considered in the next chapter.

Natural History

It is interesting to see how much of the natural history of amyloidosis in chronic paraplegia is shown by this study. It appears that up to 5 per cent of all paraplegic patients develop amyloidosis from the septic complications of spinal paralysis. The most important complication is chronic osteomyelitis from pressure sores. Chronic renal suppuration was a frequent contributory cause and, in a few patients, appeared to be the only aetiological factor. The severity and duration of the paralysis was important only in relation to the degree of septic complications. The nature of the illness causing the paraplegia was only significant when systemic illnesses that can give rise to amyloidosis in the absence of paraplegia, such as tuberculosis and some tumours, were present.

In the individual case it was impossible to predict whether amyloidosis would develop, but it was much more likely to appear when several predisposing causes were present.

The influence of amyloidosis upon the life expectancy of paraplegic patients is of practical importance. A retrospective study of the 65 cases who died with histological evidence of amyloid disease, showed development of this condition between 1·5–25 years after paraplegia with an average survival of 11·8 years. Many of these cases, however, did not receive adequate treatment by modern standards, some of them having developed their paraplegia before special centres were opened. With the advent of rectal biopsy, a safe and repeatable method of diagnosing amyloidosis is now available. Of the 15 cases that are known to have had positive rectal biopsies at Southport and Stoke Mandeville, 7 died one to three years after the first positive biopsy, and 8 are still alive, with the longest survival so far being four years. Since paraplegic patients now have a virtually normal life expectancy, unless they develop renal complications, there can be little doubt that amyloidosis has an adverse influence upon their life expectancy. This is in keeping with the views of Pidgeon (1958), Talbot (1958), Malament *et al.* (1963, 1965), and Comarr (1963). It is of practical and theoretical interest that 2 patients, 1 in this series and 1 seen subsequently, developed Wernicke's encephalopathy with mental changes, nystagmus, ataxia, and cardiac signs. The neurological features reverted to normal with intramuscular vitamin B therapy. These changes could have been due to defective absorption of the vitamin or excessive loss. Further investigations are required to elucidate the systemic effects of amyloidosis.

Once the patient has developed amyloidosis it would seem that, provided there is no severe hypertension, he can live in a fairly healthy state for a few years with a small residual renal function, as shown by the creatinine clearance, and a moderately raised blood urea. However, once the creatinine clearance falls below 20 ml/min, or the serum creatinine rises above 3 mg/100 ml, the prognosis is poor. Lethal complications that can rapidly precipitate a patient with amyloidosis into oliguric renal failure or uraemia, are episodes of dehydration, haematuria, or temporary obstruction of urine flow due to a blocked catheter or twisted condom. The primary causes of death among the 65 patients are set out in Table 6.19.

TABLE 6.19

Primary causes of death in amyloidosis and chronic paraplegia

Renal failure without hypertension	29
Renal failure with hypertension	20
Cerebro-vascular accident—secondary hypertension	5
Septicaemia with ulcerative endocarditis	3
Pneumonia	2
Myocardial infarct	1
Post-operative shock	1
Renal failure—chronic pyelonephritis (amyloidosis minimal)	1
Peritonitis—perforated gastric ulcer	1
Pulmonary tuberculosis	1
Neuroblastoma	1
	65

This study has provided much useful information about the pathology of secondary amyloidosis in paraplegia; it has shown many interesting facts concerning the distribution of amyloid within the body, and has shown how this material interferes with normal function and eventually leads to death. About two-thirds of all paraplegics who develop amyloidosis will die as a direct result of renal involvement. It will also be shown that it plays a significant part in the causation of secondary hypertension, and there is some evidence to suggest that amyloidosis may depress natural resistance to infection and allow death due to septicaemia and endocarditis to occur.

Only further clinico-pathological follow-up studies of a larger biopsy group will give the full natural history of amyloidosis and paraplegia, and show whether or not the condition is reversible.

References

ARAPAKIS, G. and TRIBE, C. R. (1963) *Ann. rheum. Dis.*, **22**, 256.
AUERBACH, O. and STEMMERMAN, M. G. (1944) *Arch. int. Med.*, **74**, 244.
BARCLAY, G. P. T., CAMERON, H. MacD. and LOUGHRIDGE, L. W. (1960) *Quart. J. Med. NS.*, **29**, 137.
BELL, E. T. (1933) *Amer. J. Path.*, **9**, 185.
BENNHOLD, H. (1923) *Dtsch. Arch. klin. Med.*, **142**, 32.
BERLYNE, S. M., VARLEY, H., NILWARANGKUR, S. and HOERNI, M. (1964) *Lancet*, ii, 874.
BLUM, A. and SOHAR, E. (1962) *Lancet*, **1**, 721.
BOWMAN, M. S. and REDFIELD, E. S. (1951) *U.S. Armed Forces Med. J.*, **2**, 715.
BORS, E., CONRAD, C. A. and MASSELL, T. B. (1954) *Surg. Gynec. Obstet.*, **99**, 451.
BOX, T. R. H. (1957) *Canad. Serv. Med. J.*, **13**, 713.
BREITHAUPT, D. J., JOUSSE, A. T. and WYNN-JONES, M. (1961) *Canad. Med. Ass. J.*, **85**, 73.
BRIGGS, G. W. (1961) *Ann. intern. Med.*, **55**, 943.
BROD, J. (1962) *Arch. Int. Pharmacodyn.*, **139**, 346.
COHEN, S. (1943) *Ann. intern. Med.*, **19**, 990.
COMARR, A. E. (1954) *Proceedings of the 3rd Annual Clinical Spinal Cord Injury Conference*, p. 30. Amer. Veterans Adm.
COMARR, A. E. (1955) *California Med.*, **82**, 332.
COMARR, A. E. (1958) *Proceedings of the 7th Annual Clinical Spinal Cord Injury Conference (Discussion)*, p. 129. Amer. Veterans Adm.
COMARR, A. E. (1963) *Proceedings of the 12th Annual Clinical Spinal Cord Injury Conference (Discussion)*, p. 40. Amer. Veterans Adm.
CONN, R. B. and SUNDBERG, R. D. (1961) *Amer. J. Path.*, **38**, 61.
DALTON, J. J., HACKLER, R. H. and BUNTS, R. C. (1965) *J. Urol.*, **93**, 553.
DICKINSON, W. H. (1877 and 1885) *On Renal and Urinary Affections*. Parts II and III. London: Longmans Green.
DIETRICK, R. B. and RUSSI, S. (1958) *J. Amer. Med. Ass.*, **166**, 41.

DOGGART, J. R., GUTTMANN, L. and SILVER, J. R. (1966) *Int. J. Paraplegia*, **3**, 229.
DUCROT, H., MONTERA, H.de., MERY, J. Ph. and RUEFF, B. (1961) *J. Urol. Nephrol. (Par.)*, **67**, 432.
FAGGE, C. H. (1876) *Trans. path. Soc. Lond.*, **27**, 324.
FENTEM, P. H., TURNBERG, L. A. and WORMSLEY, K. G. (1962) *Brit. med. J.*, **i**, 364.
FERNANDO, J. C. (1961) *J. Inst. Sci. Tech.*, **7**, 40.
GUTTMAN, P. H. (1930) *Arch. Path.*, **10**, 742, 895.
HARRISON, C. V., MILNE, M. D. and STEINER, R. E. (1956) *Quart. J. Med. NS.*, **25**, 285.
HELLER, H., MISSMAHL, H-P., SOHAR, E. and GAFNI, J. (1964) *J. Path. Bact.*, **88**, 15.
HOBBS, J. R. and MORGAN, A. D. (1963) *J. Path. Bact.*, **86**, 437.
KING, L. S. (1948) *Amer. J. Path.*, **24**, 1111.
KURBAN, A. K. (1960) *Bull. Johns Hopk. Hosp.*, **107**, 320.
LEVINE, R. A. (1962) *Amer. J. Med.*, **33**, 349.
LOUGHRIDGE, L. W. (1960) 'Renal Amyloidosis'. In *Recent Advances in Renal Disease*. London: Pitman Medical.
MACKENZIE, D. H. (1963) *Brit. med. J.*, **i**, 1449.
MAGLIO, A. and POTENZA, P. (1963) *Int. J. Paraplegia*, **1**, 131.
MALAMENT, M., FRIEDMAN, M. and PSCHIBUL, F. (1963) *Proceedings of the 12th Annual Clinical Spinal Cord Injury Conference*, p. 33. Amer. Veterans Adm.
MALAMENT, M., FRIEDMAN, M. and PSCHIBUL, F. (1965) *Arch. phys. Med.*, **46**, 406.
METCOFF, J. (1962) In *Renal Disease*, p. 267. Ed. Black, D. A. K. Oxford: Blackwell.
MCKINNEY, B. and GRUBB, CHANDRA (1965) *Nature*, **205**, 1023.
MILNE, M. D. (1962) In *Renal Disease*, p. 464. Ed. Black, D. A. K. Oxford: Blackwell.
MISSEN, G. A. K. and TRIBE, C. R. (1968) In preparation.
MISSMAHL, H-P, and GAFNI, J. (1963) *Harefuah*, **64**, 43.
MOSES, D. S. (1954) *Proceedings of the 3rd Annual Clinical Spinal Cord Injury Conference*. Amer. Veterans Adm.
NEWMAN, W. and JACOBSON, A. S. (1953) *Amer. J. Med.*, **15**, 216.
NYQUIST, R. H. (1960) *Proceedings of the 9th Annual Clinical Spinal Cord Injury Conference*, p. 109. Amer. Veterans Adm.

NYQUIST, R. H. and BORS, E. (1967) *Int. J. Paraplegia*, **5**, 22.
ORLOFF, J. and FELDER, L. (1946) *Amer. J. Med. Sci.*, **212**, 275.
PIDGEON, ITA. A. (1958) *Proceedings of the 7th Annual Clinical Spinal Cord Injury Conference*, p. 125. Amer. Veterans Adm.
PHILLIPS, R. S. (1963) *Int. J. Paraplegia*, **1**, 116.
POMERANCE, ARIELA (1966) *J. Path. Bact.*, **91**, 357.
POWELL, C. S. and SWAN, L. L. (1955) *Amer. J. Path.*, **31**, 1131.
REINGOLD, I. M. (1953) *Proceedings of the 2nd Annual Clinical Spinal Cord Injury Conference*, p. 1. Amer. Veterans Adm.
ROBINSON, R. (1954) *Proc. roy. Soc. Med.*, **47**, 1109.
ROSENBLATT, M. B. (1933) *Amer. J. Med. Sci.*, **186**, 558.
STEMMERMAN, M. G. and AUERBACH, O. (1944a) *Arch. intern. Med.*, **74**, 384.
STEMMERMAN, M. G. and AUERBACH, O. (1944b) *Amer. J. Med. Sci.*, **208**, 305.
SYMMERS, W. St., C. (1956) *J. clin. Path.*, **9**, 187.
TALBOT, H. S. (1958) *Proceedings of the 7th Annual Clinical Spinal Cord Injury Conference (Discussion)*, p. 128. Amer. Veterans Adm.
TARGGART, W. H., TRUMP, B. F., LAGUNOFF, D. and ESCHBACH, J. (1963) *Gastroenterol.*, **44**, 335.
TEILUM, G. (1964) *Acta. path. microbiol. scand.*, **61**, 21.
THOMPSON, C. E. and RICE, M. L. (1949) *Ann. intern. Med.*, **31**, 1057.
TRIBE, C. R. (1963a) *Int. J. Paraplegia*, **1**, 19, 71.
TRIBE, C. R. (1963b) *Post-mortem Findings in Paraplegic Patients*. D.M. Thesis. Oxford.
TRIBE, C. R. (1966) 'Amyloidosis in Rheumatoid Arthritis'. In *Modern Trends in Rheumatology*, p. 121. London: Butterworths.
VASQUEZ, L. E. (1963) *Arch. Collegio. Medico. de el. Salvador*, **16**, 175.
VASSAR, P. S. and CULLING, C. F. A. (1959) *Arch. Path.*, **68**, 487.
VASSAR, P. S. and CULLING, C. F. A. (1962) *Ibid.*, **73**, 71.
VILK, N. L. (1940) *Klin. Med. Mosk.*, **18**, 91.
WALKER, G. A. (1942) *Surg. Gynec. Obst.*, **75**, 374.

7

Hypertension in Chronic Paraplegia

LITTLE WORK has been published on the effects of hypertension in paraplegic patients. Reingold (1953) found the blood pressure raised in only one of 23 paraplegics who came to necropsy. This patient was found to have severe pyelonephritis and arteriosclerosis with a moderately enlarged heart. Cerebrovascular accidents are among the causes of deaths found in paraplegics by Dietrick and Russi (1958), and Nyquist (1960). The latter attributed some deaths to hypertensive encephalopathy. In a discussion after another paper by Reingold (1960), five doctors concerned with the management of paraplegics commented on the incidence of hypertension in their cases. One (Dr Bors) thought 'renal hypertension was not a rare exception in his patients', but the other four thought it exceedingly uncommon. Moeller (1962), in an investigation into the incidence and distribution of raised blood pressure in 2,223 spinal cord injury patients, concluded that these patients, who have more frequent and more severe attacks of pyelonephritis than the general population, have an incidence of diastolic hypertension not much different from the non-spinal injury population. However, examination of the figures in his article do reveal that of 138 deaths, 15 of the 36 cases with pyelonephritis had diastolic blood pressure of 90 mmHg, or higher, as compared with only 10 of the 102 cases without pyelonephritis. It was, therefore, of interest to the author (Tribe, 1963a, 1963b) to find definite clinical and pathological evidence of hypertension in 41 of the 122 patients with chronic paraplegia who came to necropsy.

Since then, Talbot (1966), in a preliminary report on *Renal Disease and Hypertension in Paraplegics and Quadriplegics*, analysed material from 43 postmortem cases. Pyelonephritis or amyloid disease, or both, were found in 35 of these. Using an arbitary definition of hypertension as a systolic pressure of 150 mmHg, or, higher, and/or diastolic pressure of 100 mmHg, or higher, he found that 16 of the 35 patients with renal disease (46%) had hypertension compared with one case (12·5%) among the remaining eight. Quadriplegics appeared to be less prone to hypertension than paraplegics. Renal disease was the cause of death in 22 patients, and of these 14 had hypertension. Of the remaining 21 patients who died of other causes, only 3 had hypertension. Hypertension developed at varying intervals after the onset of paraplegia. Commenting on these results Talbot says, 'it is difficult to escape the conviction that this is a significant difference, but equally difficult to determine precisely where the significance lies. The hypertension may reflect the severity of the disease process in the kidney, or its duration. It does not seem, in this small group, to bear any relationship to the patients age or to the presence of generalised arteriosclerosis'. The findings from our own larger series are in general agreement with the results expressed in Talbot's article.

Physiological Factors Influencing the Level of Blood Pressure in Paraplegia

Before the significance of persistently raised blood pressure in a paraplegic patient is considered, it is necessary to take into account the physiological mechanisms that regulate the blood pressure in these patients. Blood pressure is the product of the cardiac output and the peripheral resistance, and these are under the control of the sympathetic nervous system. Sympathetic stimulation causes an increase in the rate and force of contraction of the heart, and also causes vasoconstriction of the skeletal and skin arterioles and of the large veins (the capacity vessels).

The sympathetic innervation to the heart and vessels acts through different reflexes, which may be conveniently considered under three headings.

1. *Those dependent upon the medullary vasomotor centre and those mediated by mechano-receptor afferents.*

(a) Reflex vasoconstriction of the forearm blood vessels in response to the Valsalva manoeuvre.
(b) Reflex dilatation of the skin blood vessels in response to indirect heating.
(c) Reflex sweating in response to indirect heating.

2. *Those dependent upon spinal reflex arcs and independent of the vasomotor centre.*
   (a) Inspiratory vasoconstriction of the hand blood vessels (Gilliatt *et al.*, 1948).
   (b) Vasodilatation of the forearm blood vessels in response to elevation of the lower limbs (Silver, 1965).

3. *Abnormal responses not present in normal patients.* For example, autonomic hyper-reflexia in response to distension of the bladder, bowel, uterus, or other hollow viscera (Guttmann and Whitteridge, 1947). With these responses, there is a vasoconstriction of the blood vessels in the hands, accompanied by bradycardia and spells of severe hypertension.

In a low lesion, i.e. below T.12, the whole of the sympathetic nervous system is intact and there will be no difference from the normal subject in the central control of the cardiac output and the peripheral resistance. However, in lesions above T.1 (the complete tetraplegic), the whole of the sympathetic nervous system is deprived of central control from both the higher centres and the vaso-motor centre.

The abnormal responses are most marked in high cervical lesions when there is a complete interruption of the sympathetic nervous system from central control, but they are still present when a substantial part of the sympathetic is interrupted from central control and may be seen in lesions as low as T.5. The effect of complete interruption of the sympathetic in high cervical lesions is reflected in the bradycardia found at rest in tetraplegics, and it may contribute to their postural hypotension since the heart has not the same functional reserve as in the normal patient. The blood pressure is further reduced by the loss of the contraction of the capacity veins and the paralysis of the skeletal muscles, which decreases the venous return to the heart, causing a lowering of the cardiac output.

It can be readily appreciated from the foregoing remarks that an isolated reading of the blood pressure in a tetraplegic or paraplegic patient may be of little value, since if the patient has a blocked catheter or loaded rectum his blood pressure may be unduly raised. Conversely, if he is propped up, there may be an undue pooling of blood in his lower limbs, giving rise to postural hypotension, and both

these phenomena are seen very frequently in tetraplegic patients.

Sixty cases of hypertension were found in the 174 chronic paraplegics in this series, i.e. the 41 cases described in 1963 together with 19 further cases (an overall incidence of 34·8%). After describing the criteria used in the selection of these patients, the remainder of this chapter will discuss the pathological findings to show the cause of the hypertension.

Criteria of Hypertension

Because several factors affect blood pressure in paraplegics, both clinical and pathological criteria were used in the selection of these cases. Of the 60 cases finally diagnosed as hypertensive, 56 satisfied both clinical and pathological criteria, 2 were included on pathological evidence, and a further 2 on clinical evidence.

CLINICAL CRITERIA (BLOOD PRESSURE LEVELS)

From clinical notes of the 174 chronic paraplegics in this series, a record was made of all blood pressure readings. The number of such readings varied considerably and, although in the cases admitted to the Spinal Centre after 1955 an accurate clinical picture of the blood pressure level was obtained throughout their life, the majority of early cases, some of whom were injured before the opening of the National Spinal Injury Centre, had gaps of many years without blood pressure recordings. For this reason, it was only possible to establish with any accuracy the time of onset, and therefore the duration, of the hypertension in a proportion of the 60 cases. It should be noted, however, that most of these 60 cases had normal blood pressures recorded soon after the onset of their paraplegia, and they only developed a raised blood pressure in the last few years of their lives.

The limits of normal blood pressures at different ages in different sexes established by Master *et al.* (1950) were exceeded in at least one blood pressure recording during life in 58 of the 60 cases. In all but 7 cases, the diastolic pressure exceeded 100 mmHg, which Fishberg (1954) considered always pathological. He added that, 'a diastolic pressure of 95 mmHg is very suspicious and in young adults is probably abnormally high'. This latter criterion was accepted in all but 2 of the 60 cases (Table 7.1).

The effects of autonomic stimulation on the blood pressure of patients with complete lesions at T.5, and above, must be remembered when studying the blood pressure levels in paraplegics. As mentioned before, Guttmann and Whitteridge (1947) showed

TABLE 7.1

Hypertension in chronic paraplegia

Highest diastolic pressure recorded in life (60 cases)

	NO OF CASES
90–94 mmHg	2
95–100 mmHg	5
101–10 mmHg	11
111–20 mmHg	9
121–30 mmHg	6
Greater than 130 mmHg	25
No adequate recordings	2*

* These two cases were included solely on pathological evidence of hypertension.

that in such cases, on distension of the bladder or other hollow viscera, the blood pressure rose from 140/80 to between 190/130 and 250/130 and was maintained at this level for as long as the bladder pressure remained high. Hodgson and Wood (1958) repeated this work, and showed that this paroxysmal hypertension could be obliterated by ganglion blocking agents such as hexamethonium.

The levels of paraplegia in the 60 cases with hypertension in this series were—

	COMPLETE	INCOMPLETE	TOTAL
Cervical	3	2	5
Thoracic 1–5	5	1	6
Thoracic 6–12	30	5	35
Lumbar and Cauda Equina	8	4	12
Poliomyelitis		2	2

Only 11 of the 60 hypertensive cases had spinal lesions at T.5 and above. Since the blood pressure in these 11 cases might have been recorded only during periods of paroxysmal hypertension, no cases with lesions above T.6 were considered to be hypertensive without confirmatory pathological evidence. Of the total 174 chronic paraplegics in this series, 46 had spinal lesions above T.5, and the fact that only 11 (23%) were found to be hypertensive indicates that paroxysmal hypertension *per se* does not lead to cardiac hypertrophy.

The figures in this series confirm the views of Talbot (1966) that hypertension is less common in quadriplegia. Only 5 of the 28 chronic quadriplegics (18%) had hypertension in comparison with 55 of the 146 chronic paraplegics with lesions at T.1 or below (38%).

PATHOLOGICAL CRITERIA

I. Heart Weight

Fishberg (1954) considered that heart weights of more than 350 G in females, and more than 400 G in males, are highly suspicious of cardiac hypertrophy. Table 7.2 shows the recorded weights in this series.

TABLE 7.2

Heart weights in 60 cases of hypertension and chronic paraplegia

Heart weight	Death related to paraplegia (46 cases)	Death unrelated to paraplegia (14 cases)	Total
12–14 oz (335–390 G)	19	0	19
15–17 oz (420–475 G)	13	5	18
18–20 oz (505–560 G)	14	6	20
Greater than 20 oz or 560 G	0	3	3

Although in some cases the heart was near the upper limit of normality, in most cases it was definitely in excess. No other causes for cardiomegaly, apart from hypertension, were found. It has been shown in the preceeding chapter (p. 79) that when amyloid infiltration of the heart was present in chronic paraplegics, it was only found in very small amounts and could not have significantly increased the heart weight.

II. Thickness of the Left Ventricular Wall

Fishberg (1954) stated that a thickness of more than 14 mm indicated left ventricular hypertrophy. Unfortunately, no accurate measurements were made in this series, but comments on the naked-eye appearance of the left ventricle were made in all the post-mortem reports and these are shown in Table 7.3.

TABLE 7.3

*Appearance of the left ventricle in 60 cases of
hypertension and paraplegia*

	Death related to paraplegia (46)	Death unrelated to paraplegia (14)	Total
Normal thickness	2	0	2
Slight left ventricular hypertrophy	17	4	21
Moderate left ventricular hypertrophy	20	6	26
Severe left ventricular hypertrophy	7	4	11

The left ventricle was not obviously hypertrophied in only 2 cases, and these had adequate clinical evidence to justify inclusion in this series. Apart from hypertension, no other cause of left ventricular hypertrophy, such as valvular diseases of the heart, was found in this series.

Further evidence of hypertension was sought on histological grounds. The best site for such evidence is in the kidneys. In this series, however, the abundance of renal pathology unrelated to hypertension (amyloidosis and pyelonephritis) made it impossible, unless malignant nephrosclerosis was present, to be certain whether or not the renal vascular changes were due to hypertension. Similarly, when examining the vessels in other organs the histological picture was often obscured by amyloid infiltration.

Analysis of Cases, with Discussion Concerning the Pathological Effects and Likely Cause of Hypertension in Paraplegia

The 60 cases of hypertension established by these criteria fell into two groups, on separating them into those who had died from causes related and unrelated to their paraplegia (Table 7.4).

Table 7.4 shows a high incidence of hypertension in the chronic paraplegics in this post-mortem series (34·8%). This figure is comparable with those obtained by Moeller (1962), 41·7 per cent, and Talbot (1966), 40 per cent, both derived from smaller numbers of cases.

The younger age group had a high incidence of cerebro-vascular accidents, malignant hypertension, terminal uraemia, pericarditis, amyloidosis, and chronic pyelonephritis. The older group showed few serious complications of hypertension, but had a high incidence of severe coronary atheroma.

The variables (1–8) listed in Table 7.4 will be discussed further, both to describe the pathological effects of hypertension and to try to understand the cause of the hypertension in this series.

Age

The first obvious difference between these two groups was the average age at death. A breakdown of the ages at death is shown in Table 7.5.

Nearly all authors consider hypertension in young persons to be secondary. Platt (1948) studied severe hypertension in young persons and included 66 cases of secondary hypertension with an average age of 39·5 years (19 of whom were under thirty-five). Heptinstall (1953), in his survey of 51 cases of

TABLE 7.4

Hypertension in chronic paraplegia

	Death related to paraplegia (117 cases)	Death unrelated to paraplegia (57 cases)	Total (174)
NO. WITH HYPERTENSION	46 (39·4%)	14 (24·3%)	60 (34·8%)
1. Average age at death in years	39·4	54·2	42·8
2. Cerebrovascular accidents	6	1	7
3. Malignant hypertension	8	1	9
4. Blood urea above 200 mg per cent at death	29	1	30
5. Severe coronary atheroma at death	1	7	8
6. Uraemic pericarditis at death	13	0	13
7. Associated amyloidosis	29	2	31
8. Severe chronic pyelonephritis at death	21	0	21

TABLE 7.5
Hypertension in chronic paraplegia (Ages at death in 60 cases)

	Death related to paraplegia (46 cases)	Death unrelated to paraplegia (14 cases)	Total
Up to 30 years	2	0	2
30–34 years	13	0	13
35–40 years	14	1	15
41–45 years	9	2	11
More than 45 years	8	11	19

malignant hypertension, found no cases of primary hypertension below the age of thirty-five. Therefore, on age alone, the patients who died from causes related to their paraplegia would be expected to have secondary hypertension. Since most cases in this group had chronic kidney disease and none had any other causes of secondary hypertension (e.g. phaeochromocytoma, endocrine causes, etc.), the secondary hypertension appears to have been of renal origin.

Cerebrovascular Accidents

Some comments about the part played by cerebrovascular accidents in the causes of death of paraplegics have already been made in Chapter 2 (p. 4). Seven patients died from massive haemorrhages, and details are shown in Table 7.6.

Although 4 of these cases had amyloidosis, no evidence of amyloid deposition in the walls of the cerebral vessels was found in this series, and there

was no evidence of any local cause for the cerebral haemorrhages. Atheroma, both of the coronary and cerebral vessels, was either slight or absent in all cases and hypertension was the only causative agent in these cerebrovascular accidents. Malignant hypertension was confirmed in only one case. The nature of the hypertension is not easy to establish. Two patients, with C.8/T.1 and T.3 lesions, were liable to paroxysmal hypertension. However, only one cerebral haemorrhage was attributed to this cause in a large number of cervical and upper thoracic cases, and this patient (described in detail in Chapter 2, p. 4) showed no clinical or pathological evidence of sustained hypertension.

Only one case (No. 171) had no significant renal disease, and at the age of fifty-two his hypertension was probably essential in nature. The remaining 6 cases all showed extensive chronic renal disease: 2 had severe chronic pyelonephritis; 3 chronic pyelonephritis with amyloidosis; and one severe renal amyloidosis without pyelonephritis. All 6 developed their hypertension after their paraplegia, and in the 4 patients who were aged forty or below at the time of their death the hypertension was almost certainly secondary to chronic renal disease. The aetiology in the other 2 cases, aged fifty-one and fifty-five at death, is more debatable, but as they had extensive renal disease they were considered to have died from causes related to their paraplegia.

Malignant Hypertension

Only 2 patients had a definite clinical diagnosis of malignant hypertension made during life, but pathological changes showed that the hypertension in 9 patients had progressed to the malignant phase. The early German writers on the pathological diagnosis of malignant hypertension were followed by the classical paper of Kimmelstiel and Wilson

TABLE 7.6
Cerebrovascular accidents in chronic paraplegics with hypertension

Case no.	Age at death	Level of spinal lesion	Coronary atheroma	Chronic pyelo-nephritis	Amyloidosis Grade in body	Grade in kidneys	Evidence of malignant hypertension
45	36	C.8/T.1	−	+ +	II	+ + +	Doubtful
54	39	Cauda equina	−	+ + +	I	+	No
61	40	T.12	−	+ + +	—	—	Yes
143	51	T.3	+	+ + + (unilateral)	III	+ + +	No
156	32	T.7	±	Nil	II	+ + +	No
210	55	T.11	±	+ + + +	—	—	No
171	52	L.1	±	±	—	—	No

8

(1936) and, more recently, by the excellent papers of Heptinstall (1953, 1966) and Kincaid-Smith *et al.* (1958). From study of these and other papers it was decided to adhere to the criteria laid down by Heptinstall. These can be summarised as—

Absolute criteria. 1. Glomerular tuft necrosis leading to crescent formation and glomerulitis in 50 per cent or less of the glomeruli.
2. Fibrinoid necrosis of the renal arterioles.

Confirmatory criteria. 3. Evidence of fibrinoid necrosis in extra-renal vessels.
4. Collagenous intimal proliferation of the interlobular renal arteries ('Endarteritis fibrosa').

Endarteritis fibrosa was so frequently found in the focal lesions of chronic pyelonephritis (Fig. 7.1 and *see* Fig. 5.14), unassociated with fibrinoid necrosis of the arterioles or glomerulitis, that it was not considered pathognomic of malignant hypertension.

combination of renal amyloidosis and malignant hypertension is illustrated in Fig. 7.2 and 7.3. Brief clinical and pathological details of the 9 cases are presented in Table 7.7 (p. 98).

Table 7.7 shows that—

1. In agreement with other authors, the ages of these patients tend to be lower than those with benign hypertension. (Average age at death 38·9 years.)
2. All cases occurred in patients with spinal lesions below T.5, so paroxysmal hypertension played no part in their pathogenesis.
3. Only one case had any evidence of significant coronary atheroma.
4. As found by other authors (Heptinstall, 1966) the diastolic pressures were all 130 mmHg or over, and rose as high as 180 mmHg in 2 patients.
5. All patients had terminal uraemia. One patient (No. 61), with a level of 122 mg per cent, died from a massive cerebral haemorrhage and in another patient (No. 195), in whom the level was 105 mg per cent, hypertensive encephalopathy and cardiac failure played the major part in the cause of death. In the remaining 7 patients the blood

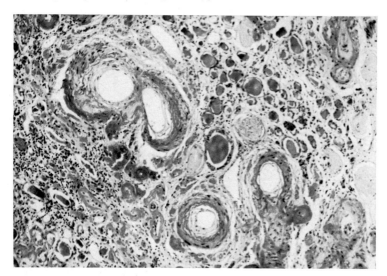

FIG. 7.1. Vascular changes in chronic pyelonephritis. Note the marked 'endarteritis fibrosa' with reduplication of the internal elastic laminae in a group of medium-sized renal arteries, in an area of atrophic chronic pyelonephritis. There is also early infiltration of the vessel walls by amyloid. H & E. ×108. Case no. 143. For details of case-history see p. 15.

The pathological diagnosis of malignant hypertension was often made more difficult by the presence of amyloid. This tended to obscure the vascular changes, and it was often impossible to distinguish with certainty the presence of true fibrinoid necrosis in the vessels and glomerular tufts. However, in spite of severe renal amyloidosis, there were some cases in which glomerulitis and crescent formation could be distinguished and in these patients the diagnosis of malignant hypertension was made purely on this one histological finding. This unusual

urea levels ranged at death from 165 to 535 mg per cent. Although chronic renal disease was frequently present in these patients, the malignant nephrosclerosis undoubtedly accelerated the eventual failure.

6. All the cases had some chronic pyelonephritis, but in only 3 was this severe and in 2 of these there was only unilateral involvement.
7. Severe or moderate renal amyloidosis was present in 5 cases and, in at least 3, this appeared to be the predominant chronic renal disease.

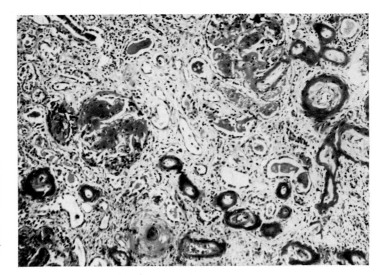

FIG. 7.2. Malignant hypertension and amyloidosis. Case no. 97. The renal glomeruli are partially replaced by amyloid and in one glomerulus there is early, but definite, glomerulitis with 'crescent' formation, The severe infiltration of the vessel walls by amyloid obscures any evidence of fibrinoid necrosis. H & E. ×120.

8. In probably all these cases the hypertension was secondary to chronic renal disease, and, in all but one, this was directly related to their paraplegia. In the last case (no. 180), a complete paraplegia below T.10 occurred in a forty-two year old male Nigerian after an aortogram performed at another hospital for the investigation of severe hypertension. He died four years later from renal failure, and necropsy showed extensive fibrinoid necrosis in the renal arterioles and pancreatic vessels, with a localised area of chronic pyelonephritis in the upper pole of the right kidney. Some Schistosoma ova embedded deep in the wall of the bladder provided the clue to the probable sequence of events.

9. As mentioned before, the most common histological criteria of malignant hypertension in these cases was glomerular tuft necrosis, leading to crescent formation and glomerulitis, and this could sometimes be distinguished in spite of severe renal amyloidosis. Photomicrographs from some of these cases are shown in Figs. 7.2 and 7.3.

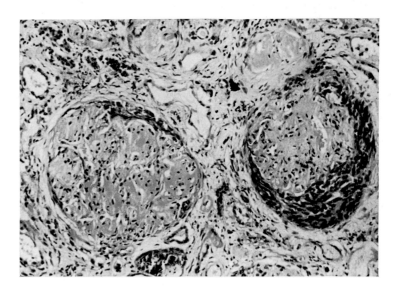

FIG. 7.3. Malignant hypertension and amyloidosis. Case no. 211. The renal glomeruli are nearly replaced by amyloid and there is marked proliferative glomerulitis and 'crescent' formation. H & E. ×250.

TABLE 7.7

Malignant hypertension in chronic paraplegia

Case no.	Age	Level of spinal lesion	Coronary atheroma	Highest BP in life	Terminal blood urea mg%	CPN*	Amyloid Grade in body	Grade in kidneys	Histological criteria of malignant hypertension (details p. 96)
43	39	T.11	±	250/180	235	+	—	—	Criteria 1 and 3
61	40	T.12	—	240/145	122	+ + +	—	—	Criteria 1
97	30	T.8	+	220/140	565	+	I	+ +	Criteria 1 and 2
138	41	C/E	+	240/170	320	+	—	—	Criteria 1, 2, and 3
173	31	T.6	+	230/180	165	+ + Unilateral	II	+ + +	Criteria 1
195	45	T.11	±	260/170	105	+ + + + Unilateral	I	+ + +	Criteria 1
202	42	L.2	+ +	230/140	472	+	II	+ + +	Criteria 1
211	41	L.3	+	220/130	300	+	II	+ + +	Criteria 1
180	46	T.10	+	280/155	535	+	—	—	Criteria 2 and 3

*CPN = Chronic pyelonephritis.

Renal Failure

In the group of hypertensive patients who died from causes related to their paraplegia, a high proportion died from renal failure. Of the 46 patients, 29 had a terminal blood urea greater than 200 mg per cent, and in a further 11 cases the blood urea was between 100–200 mg per cent. This is in contrast to the smaller group of hypertensive patients who died from causes unrelated to their paraplegia. Among the latter, only 2 of 14 had terminal blood urea levels greater than 100 mg per cent. One of these was the case of malignant hypertension described before (p. 97), and the other was a man of fifty-three who died from myocardial infarction due to severe coronary atheroma. He had had moderate hypertension for the last ten of his twenty-four years as a paraplegic. His terminal blood urea of 110 mg per cent was apparently related to a bilateral renal vein thrombosis and moderate renal amyloidosis found at necropsy. (Further details in Table 6.9, p. 71.)

The part that hypertension played in the cause of renal failure in this series is complex, but there is little doubt that where present it contributed to the rate of destruction of renal tissue. These figures, however, add considerable support to the view that in most cases the hypertension was secondary to chronic renal disease.

Coronary Heart Disease

Weiss and Parker, in their paper on pyelonephritis in 1939, noted that thrombosis or haemorrhage of the cerebral arteries, and coronary disease, rarely occurred in their cases of pyelonephritis associated with hypertension. It might be thought that the immobility of the paraplegic would lead to obesity and, thus, a high incidence of coronary atheroma. However, in our series no such findings were noted. Table 7.8 shows the overall incidence of coronary atheroma among the chronic paraplegics.

The relationship of coronary atheroma to hypertension is complex, and the higher incidence of severe coronary atheroma found among the small group of older hypertensives dying from causes unrelated to their paraplegia is presumably a reflection of the general increase in atheroma which occurs with ageing.

TABLE 7.8

Coronary atheroma in chronic paraplegia

Degree of coronary atheroma	Death related to paraplegia (117 cases)	Death unrelated to paraplegia (57 cases)	Totals (174 cases)
Nil	59 (30)*	27 (5)*	86 (35)*
Slight	29 (11)	16 (1)	45 (12)
Moderate	17 (4)	3 (1)	20 (5)
Severe	12 (1)	11 (7)	23 (8)

* The figures in brackets indicate the number in each group occurring in cases with hypertension.

Uraemic Pericarditis

Of the 86 patients who died from renal failure due to causes related to their paraplegia, 19 (22%) had uraemic pericarditis, and of these 13 had hypertension (3 in the malignant phase). *See* Fig. 7.4.

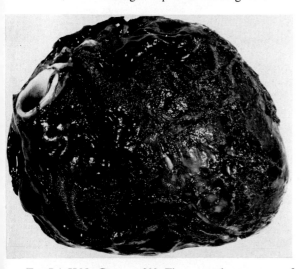

FIG. 7.4. H.N., Case no. 202. The external appearance of the heart of a forty-four year old paraplegic who died twenty years after a complete paralysis below L.2 from a gunshot wound. Death was due to renal failure from malignant hypertension secondary to renal amyloidosis and mild chronic pyelonephritis. There is a confluent haemorrhagic fibrinous 'uraemic' type of pericarditis.

These figures differ considerably from those in the literature. Hopps and Wissler (1955) described 107 patients who died in uraemia and found uraemic pericarditis in 60 (56%). Kimmelstiel *et al.* (1961) found only 22 cases of pericarditis in 100 patients dying in uraemia, and considered that uraemic pericarditis was rare without hypertension. Our figures are in general agreement with their findings. Kincaid-Smith *et al.* (1958) described 124 cases of malignant hypertension and found the overall incidence of fibrinous pericarditis was 21 per cent.

The part played by hypertension in the development of uraemic pericarditis is still so little understood that the findings in this series, though of interest, add little to an understanding of the causes of their hypertension.

Amyloidosis and Hypertension

It has been frequently noted that the incidence of hypertension in amyloidosis is low, and some authors have stated that renal amyloidosis is the only chronic renal disease not associated with hypertension. As early as 1877, Howship Dickinson noted the general absence of hypertrophy of the heart with lardaceous disease and found only 6 instances in 83 cases. Table 7.9 shows the incidence found by several authors.

TABLE 7.9

Hypertension and amyloidosis

Authors	Cases	No. of hypertensives
Rosenblatt, 1933	110	0
Bell, 1933	65	6
Dixon, 1934	100	4
Altnow *et al.*, 1939	57	Very infrequent
Cohen, 1943	79	8
Auerbach and Stemmerman, 1944	144	3
Dahlin, 1949	30	1
Zuckerbod *et al.*, 1956	39	8
Heptinstall and Joekes, 1960	11	6

Leard and Jacques (1950) reported a man with secondary amyloidosis due to osteomyelitis. He had hypertension (blood pressure 180/130) and died at the age of twenty-four. At necropsy, the kidneys were contracted but showed only severe amyloidosis. These authors reviewed the literature and could find only 39 cases of previously reported amyloidosis and hypertension. In only 9 of these was there an adequate description of the kidney pathology, and in most the kidneys were contracted.

Heptinstall and Joekes (1960) in a report of 11 cases of renal amyloid proven by renal biopsy, found that 6 had hypertension (diastolic pressure greater than 100 mmHg). They attributed this high incidence to the general well-being of their patients in comparison to the large series reported in the 1930s and 1940s, the majority of whom had tuberculosis combined with amyloidosis. The suggestion that involvement of the adrenals by amyloid may cause hypotension in these patients, is largely ruled out by the extreme rarity of Addison's disease from this cause (Guttman, 1930; Stemmerman and Auerbach, 1944; and our own findings). Hypertension appears to be more common in primary amyloidosis. Marietta (1962) found 70 cases in the literature, and considered that the hypertension did not correlate with the extent of renal amyloidosis, nutritional state, or adrenal involvement.

Of the 65 cases of amyloidosis in chronic paraplegia in this series, it was of interest to note that 31 (48%) had clinical and pathological evidence of hypertension. Table 7.10 shows the incidence and degree of chronic renal disease in these patients.

TABLE 7.10
Amyloidosis and hypertension in chronic paraplegia

Incidence and degree of chronic renal disease (31 cases)*
Average age at death 39·7 years

CHRONIC PYELONEPHRITIS		RENAL AMYLOIDOSIS	
Nil	4 cases	+	4 cases
±	3 cases	+ +	6 cases
+	10 cases	+ + +	21 cases
+ +	4 cases		
+ + +	10 cases		

* The figures for chronic pyelonephritis and renal amyloidosis are not comparable.

A detailed study of the individual cases showed that in a few, aged over fifty at death, the hypertension was probably essential in type. The majority were aged under forty at death and had a mixture of chronic pyelonephritis and renal amyloidosis. Of these, 14 had severe or moderate chronic pyelonephritis, but there was a larger group with severe renal amyloidosis and only mild chronic pyelonephritis (grades ± and +), and in 2 cases, aged thirty-two and thirty-four at death, severe renal amyloidosis was present with no evidence of chronic pyelonephritis. It should be pointed out that the histological changes of chronic pyelonephritis were not destroyed or obscured by subsequent renal amyloidosis. Although in most of these cases the hypertension was probably secondary to chronic pyelonephritis, renal amyloidosis played a large part in causing the hypertension in a few cases and a contributory part in a significant number.

Chronic Pyelonephritis

The relationship of pyelonephritis to hypertension is still not fully understood. Although a few writers believe that there is no relationship (Pearman *et al.*, 1940; Goldring and Chasis, 1944), the majority believe that the incidence of hypertension is significantly higher in patients with chronic pyelonephritis (Weiss and Parker, 1939; Braasch *et al.*, 1940; Brod, 1956; Robertson *et al.*, 1962). Chronic pyelonephritis is also frequently quoted as a cause of malignant hypertension (Heptinstall, 1953; Kincaid-Smith *et al.*, 1955). Some authors go so far as to state that, in the overwhelming majority of cases, chronic pyelonephritis is the cause of malignant hypertension (Saphir and Taylor, 1952; Saphir, 1961). Other authors prefer to be uncommitted. Kleeman *et al.* (1960), in a most comprehensive review of pyelonephritis, only go so far as to state that pyelonephritis can exacerbate and intensify a pre-existing hypertension, regardless of how mild it is.

The mechanism by which pyelonephritis causes hypertension is also the subject of considerable discussion. Kincaid-Smith (1955) postulated that ischaemic areas (incomplete infarcts), produced as a result of arteritis secondary to infection, were the underlying cause. However, recent experimental work by Heptinstall *et al.* (1960) and Alexander *et al.* (1961) has shown that chronic pyelonephritis may develop without any arterial lesions, and also that ischaemic areas do not always result in hypertension.

The only unequivocal evidence that a renal lesion such as chronic pyelonephritis can cause hypertension in man, is the permanent relief of hypertension by nephrectomy for unilateral renal disease. Barker and Walters (1940) and Pickering and Heptinstall (1953) were among the first authors to quote cases with unilateral pyelonephritis who were 'cured' by nephrectomy and had remained normotensive after a number of years.

Pickering (1955) stated that chronic pyelonephritis seemed to offer an unusual opportunity for deciding what, in man, is the nature of the renal factor which causes hypertension. He further stressed the need for information as to the incidence of different levels of arterial pressure in an unselected series of cases of chronic pyelonephritis, and data relating their blood pressure levels to other clinical features.

In many ways the present series satisfies the above requirements. First, and most important, the patients presented as a group with chronic pyelonephritis selected only because of their paraplegia, and the incidence of hypertension was established later. Second, there is little doubt about the pathological diagnosis of pyelonephritis; a cause of argument in other series. Too many articles on this subject have run into difficulties because they have been written in the wrong order, i.e. cases of hypertension were studied to see how many had chronic pyelonephritis. Third, there is adequate clinical and pathological data available. The objections to the findings in this series are the presence of mixed renal pathology and the possible specific relationship of hypertension to paraplegia. These points have been discussed elsewhere and do not affect the findings concerning chronic pyelonephritis and hypertension in this series.

the hypertensive from the non-hypertensive cases unless there were changes due to malignant nephrosclerosis.

On the other hand, only 4 of the 26 patients who died from causes related to their paraplegia, with chronic pyelonephritis graded $++$, developed hypertension. Of these 4 patients, 3 had severe focal atrophic chronic pyelonephritis, and one active chronic pyelonephritis. This last patient was included as he died from a cerebral haemorrhage, with one recorded blood pressure of 170/100 and a slightly

TABLE 7.11
Hypertension in chronic paraplegia

Incidence of chronic pyelonephritis

Degree of chronic pyelonephritis	Death related to paraplegia		Death unrelated to paraplegia		Totals	
	All cases	Hypertensives	All cases	Hypertensives	All cases	Hypertensives
Nil	13	4*	21	3	34	7
± and +	30	15	18	8	48	23
++	26	4	13	2	39	6
+++	35	21	2	0	37	21
No histology available	13	2	3	1	16	3
Totals	117	46	57	14	174	60

* These four cases had pure renal amyloidosis.

The evidence presented in Table 7.4, and amplified since, indicates that there is a large group of young secondary hypertensives in this series. It is probable that in most cases the hypertension was due to chronic pyelonephritis, and further details of this association are given in Table 7.11.

Before drawing any conclusions from Table 7.11, it must be recalled that a $+++$ grading for pyelonephritis was only made in cases of generalised atrophic chronic pyelonephritis, and the grading $++$ usually was made in cases of widespread focal active chronic pyelonephritis (*see* p. 46 for further details).

Of the 35 patients who died from causes related to their paraplegia, with chronic pyelonephritis graded $+++$, 21 developed hypertension. It appears therefore, that although widespread atrophic chronic pyelonephritis was frequently associated with hypertension, this was not invariable. Although the kidneys from these cases were studied with care, it was impossible on histological grounds to distinguish

enlarged heart (13 oz). Most of the 22 non-hypertensives in this group had active chronic pyelonephritis. From this relatively small series, it seems that hypertension usually develops when the chronic pyelonephritis has progressed to the atrophic, or 'healing', phase and rarely occurs when the disease is still in the active phase.

Of the 30 patients who died from causes related to their paraplegia, with either ± or + chronic pyelonephritis, 15 had hypertension. Of these, 2 had malignant hypertension without amyloidosis and the remainder had associated severe renal amyloidosis. As discussed on p. 100, it is probable that the renal amyloid played a large part in the aetiology of the hypertension in this group.

Only 4 patients, among those who died from causes related to their paraplegia, had 'pure renal amyloidosis' with no evidence of chronic pyelonephritis. In 2 of these, aged thirty-two and thirty-four at death, the amyloid was thought to be the cause of their hypertension. One patient, aged sixty-one at death, could have developed essential hypertension. The fourth patient was a man, aged thirty-four at death, who had lived twelve years after an incomplete traumatic paraplegia at C.6. He had severe pressure sores with underlying osteomyelitis, and was hypertensive for the last year and a half of his life. He died from renal failure and at post-mortem had a uraemic pericarditis, enlarged heart (17 oz), but no coronary atheroma. His kidneys were enlarged and joined by their lower poles to form a classical horseshoe kidney (*see* Fig. 6.5). On microscopy, this showed 'pure renal amyloidosis' and, although there was a terminal unilateral pyonephrosis there was no evidence of chronic pyelonephritis. His hypertension could be attributed to pure renal amyloidosis, but it is well known that congenital lesions of the kidneys are often associated with secondary hypertension and this case must remain not proven.

TO SUMMARISE

From the evidence presented, there seems little doubt that most of the 46 patients with hypertension, in the 117 chronic paraplegics who died from causes related to their paraplegia, developed high blood pressure secondary to chronic renal disease. The exact nature of their underlying renal pathology was difficult to determine, but Table 7.12 shows the likely aetiology factors.

In contrast, 14 cases of hypertension were found among the 57 chronic paraplegics who died from causes unrelated to their paraplegia, and in only 2 was the hypertension probably secondary to renal disease. The first was in a man aged thirty-six at death, who died from respiratory failure due to chronic spinal meningitis and at necropsy had a grossly enlarged heart (21 oz) with a diffuse subacute glomerulonephritis that had been present

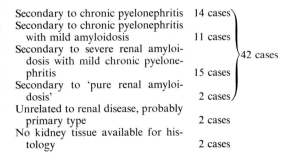

TABLE 7.12

Aetiology of hypertension in chronic paraplegia

Patients who died from causes related to their Paraplegia (46)

Secondary to chronic pyelonephritis	14 cases
Secondary to chronic pyelonephritis with mild amyloidosis	11 cases
Secondary to severe renal amyloidosis with mild chronic pyelonephritis	15 cases
Secondary to 'pure renal amyloidosis'	2 cases
Unrelated to renal disease, probably primary type	2 cases
No kidney tissue available for histology	2 cases

(14, 11, 15, 2 cases braced together = 42 cases)

before the paraplegia. The second was the patient discussed before (p. 97), who died from renal failure with malignant hypertension that developed before his paraplegia and was probably secondary to chronic pyelonephritis related to urinary schistosomiasis. Although in the remaining 12 cases in this group most showed slight or moderate chronic pyelonephritis, and there were 2 cases of renal amyloidosis, these were in a much older age group and the hypertension was probably primary.

Therefore, of the 60 cases of hypertension in this series it is thought that at least 44 (73%) developed hypertension secondary to chronic renal disease, and in 42 (70%) the renal pathology was directly related to the septic complications of paraplegia.

The Part Played by Hypertension in the Causes of Death in Chronic Paraplegia

The hypertension in these patients contributed to death in one or more of three ways, by its association with—

1. Cerebrovascular accidents
2. Renal failure
3. Cardiac failure.

In fatal cerebral haemorrhage it was clear that the hypertension played the major part in causing death.

In most patients who died in uraemia, the mixed renal pathology obscured the part played by hypertension in causing renal failure. Renal failure could be attributed solely to high blood pressure only in those cases with histological evidence of malignant hypertension. In the remaining cases, the hypertension was thought to have contributed to the cause of death.

Some patients died with signs of hypertensive heart failure and many showed bilateral pleural effusions and pulmonary oedema at post-mortem. These signs were difficult to interpret, as they often occurred in patients who died from renal failure without hypertension.

Taking these difficulties into consideration, the

final assessment of the part played by hypertension in the 117 chronic paraplegics who died from causes related to their paraplegia is—

1. Hypertension the major cause of death: 20 cases.
2. Hypertension a contributory cause of death: 19 cases.
3. Hypertension present, but played no significant part in the cause of death: 7 cases.

References

ALEXANDER, N., HEPTINSTALL, R. H. and PICKERING, G. W. (1961) *J. Path. Bact.*, **81**, 225.
ALTNOW, H. O., VAN WINKLE, C. C. and COHEN, S. S. (1939) *Arch. int. Med.*, **63**, 249.
AUERBACH, O. and STEMMERMAN, M. G. (1944) *Arch. int. Med.*, **74**, 244.
BARKER, N. W. and WALTERS, W. (1940) *Proc. staff Meet. Mayo Clinic*, **15**, 475.
BELL, E. T. (1933) *Amer. J. Path.*, **9**, 185.
BRAASCH, W. F., WALTERS, W. and HAMMER, H. J. (1940) *Proc. staff Meet. Mayo Clinic*, **15**, 477.
BROD, J. (1956) *Lancet*, **i**, 973.
COHEN, S. (1943) *Ann. intern. Med.*, **19**, 990.
DAHLIN, D. C. (1949) *Proc. staff Meet. Mayo Clinic*, **24**, 637.
DICKINSON, W. H. (1877) *The Pathology and Treatment of Albuminuria*, 2nd ed., Chapters 11–13. London: Longmans Green.
DIETRICK, R. B. and RUSSI, S. (1958) *J. Amer. Med. Ass.*, **166**, 41.
DIXON, H. M. (1934) *Amer. J. Med. Sci.*, **187**, 401.
FISHBERG, A. M. (1954) *Hypertension and Nephritis*. London: Ballière, Tindall & Cox.
GILLIATT, R. W., GUTTMANN, L. and WHITTERIDGE, D. (1948) *J. Physiol.*, **107**, 67.
GOLDRING, W. and CHASIS, H. (1944) *Hypertension and Hypertensive Disease*. New York: The Commonwealth Fund.
GUTTMAN, P. H. (1930) *Arch. Path.*, **10**, 742 and 895.
GUTTMANN, L. and WHITTERIDGE, D. (1947) *Brain*, **70**, 361.
HEPTINSTALL, R. H. (1953) *J. Path. Bact.*, **65**, 423.
HEPTINSTALL, R. H. (1960) *Recent Advances in Pathology*, 7th ed., Chapter 4. London: J. & A. Churchill.
HEPTINSTALL, R. H. (1966) *Pathology of the Kidney*. Boston: Little, Brown.
HEPTINSTALL, R. H. and JOEKES, A. M. (1960) *Ann. Rheum. Dis.*, **19**, 126.
HODGSON, N. B. and WOOD, J. A. (1958) *J. Urol.*, **79**, 719.
HOPPS, H. C. and WISSLER, R. W. (1955) *Amer. J. Path.*, **31**, 261.
KIMMELSTIEL, P. and WILSON, C. (1936) *Amer. J. Path.*, **12**, 45.
KIMMELSTIEL, P., KIM, O. J., BERES, J. A. and WELLMANN, K. (1961) *Amer. J. Med.*, **30**, 589.
KINCAID-SMITH, PRISCILLA, (1955) *Lancet*, **ii**, 1263.
KINCAID-SMITH, P., MCMICHAEL, J. and MURPHY, E. A. (1958) *Quart. J. Med. N.S.*, **27**, 117.
KLEEMAN, C. R., HEWITT, W. L. and GUZE, L. B. (1960) *Medicine (Baltimore)*, **39**, 3.
LEARD, S. E. and JAQUES, W. E. (1950) *New Engl. J. Med.*, **242**, 891.
MARIETTA, J. S. (1962) *Southern Med. J.*, **55**, 374.
MASTER, A. M., DUBLIN, L. I. and MARKS, H. H. (1950) *J. Amer. Med. Ass.*, **143**, 1464.
MOELLER, B. A. Jr. (1958) *Proceedings of the 7th Annual Clinical Spinal Cord Injury Conference*, p. 1. Amer. Veterans Adm.
NYQUIST, R. H. (1960) *Proceedings of the 9th Annual Clinical Spinal Cord Injury Conference*, p. 109. Amer. Veterans Adm.
PEARMEN, R. O., THOMPSON, G. J. and ALLEN, E. V. (1940) *Proc. staff Meet. Mayo Clinic*, **15**, 467.
PICKERING, G. W. (1955) *High Blood Pressure*. London: Churchill.
PICKERING, G. W. and HEPTINSTALL, R. H. (1953) *Quart. J. Med. N.S.*, **22**, 1.
PLATT, R. (1948) *Quart. J. Med. N.S.*, **17**, 83.
REINGOLD, I. M. (1953) *Proceedings of the 2nd Annual Clinical Spinal Cord Injury Conference*, p. 1. Amer. Veterans Adm.
REINGOLD, I. M. (1960) *Proceedings of the 9th Annual Clinical Spinal Cord Injury Conference*, p. 112. Amer. Veterans Adm.
ROBERTSON, P. W., KLIDJIAN, A., HULL, D. H., HILTON, D. D. and DYSON, M. L. (1962) *Lancet*, **ii**, 567.
ROSENBLATT, M. B. (1933) *Amer. J. Med. Sci.*, **186**, 558.
SAPHIR, O. (1961) *Southern Med. J.*, **54**, 834.
SAPHIR, O. and TAYLOR, B. (1952) *Ann. int. Med.*, **36**, 1017.
SILVER, J. R. (1965) *Int. J. Paraplegia*, **4**, 235.
TALBOT, H. S. (1966) *Med. Serv. J. Canada*, **22**, 570.
TRIBE, C. R. (1963a) *Int. J. Paraplegia*, **1**, 19.
TRIBE, C. R. (1963b) *Post-mortem Findings in Paraplegic Patients*. D.M. Thesis. Oxford.
WEISS, S. and PARKER, F. (1939) *Medicine (Baltimore)*, **18**, 221.
ZUCKERBOD, M., ROSENBERG, B. and KAYDEN, H. J. (1956) *Amer. J. Med.*, **21**, 227.

Index